GETTING to Baby

Creating your Family
Faster, Easier, and
Less Expensive
Through Fertility,
Adoption or Surrogacy

Victoria Collier & Jennifer Collier

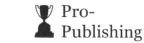

Pro-
Publishing
an imprint of Morgan James Publishing
NEW YORK

GETTING TO Baby

Creating your Family Faster, Easier, and Less Expensive
Through Fertility, Adoption or Surrogacy

by **Victoria Collier & Jennifer Collier**

© 2011 Victoria Collier & Jennifer Collier. All rights reserved.

ISBN 978-0-98285-909-4 (paperback)

Published by:

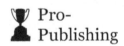

Pro-Publishing

an imprint of

MORGAN JAMES PUBLISHING
The Entrepreneurial Publisher
5 Penn Plaza, 23rd Floor
New York City, New York 10001
(212) 655-5470 Office
(516) 908-4496 Fax
www.MorganJamesPublishing.com

Cover Design by:
Rachel Lopez
rachel@r2cdesign.com

Interior Design by:
Bonnie Bushman
bbushman@bresnan.net

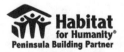

In an effort to support local communities, raise awareness and funds, Morgan James Publishing donates one percent of all book sales for the life of each book to Habitat for Humanity.
Get involved today, visit
www.HelpHabitatForHumanity.org.

Dedication

We lovingly dedicate this book to our children,

Katherine and Christopher.

Acknowledgements

Our children, our joy, and this book would not have been possible without the love shared by others.

We specifically want to thank and acknowledge our surrogate, Brittany, who gave of herself selflessly and who endured such a difficult pregnancy. Words are not adequate to express just how grateful we are. We, as well as the children, will always love you.

A special "thank you" to Mike Prieto for sharing his surrogacy experience with us. Without the willingness of others to share their pain as well as their joy, we would have never known about or considered surrogacy.

Our journey was a long one and we had many loving supporters travel it with us. We thank our friends and family who were strong and supportive of us as when we lost our child, had two failed adoptions, and ultimately celebrated the birth of our children. We know it was emotional for all involved and we could not have done it without you.

What Others are Saying About

Getting to Baby

"As an adoptive parent and an adoption attorney for over 35 years, I find that my clients have so many questions about how to create their families and are interested in what experiences other couples have had. **Getting to Baby** *shares the personal experiences of Victoria and Jennifer—through disappointment to success. It tells it like it was for them and includes very practical pointers that can be helpful to others. The authors became champions of surrogacy and encourage others to be successful in creating their families. A must read for anyone experiencing challenges in creating their family."*

—**James B. Outman,** Fellow of the American Academy of Adoption Attorneys, Fellow of the Georgia Council of Adoption Lawyers, Law Office of James B. Outman, LLC, Atlanta, GA

*"**Getting to Baby** provides a unique and fresh approach to creating a family. Victoria and Jennifer Collier share their vulnerabilities sincerely to guide others through their own journey to have a family. After having gone through my own process—International Adoption—I can say with certainty that I would have benefited by having and reading this book before and during my own journey. This is such* an important and beautiful *story to help others see through many different options."*

—**Susan Kovac Sanders**, CRNA, Mother of John Gray Timur Sanders (adopted from Russia, 2009)

Table of Contents

Author's Note and Disclosure:...xi
Baby's Face..1

CHAPTER 1 Preparing to Create Your Family Now 3

Where is Your Mind? *3*
Getting On The Same Page: The Importance of Communication,
Care-Giving and Setting a Budget *5*
Set a Budget...*6*
It's Not a Perfect World..*7*
Discussing Alternatives With Each Other *8*
Have a Support Team *9*

Getting to Baby: Communication Story 9

Finding Support Through Social Media: Facebook........................*11*
Different Strokes for Different Folks: The Importance of a Positive
Attitude and Self-Care *11*
Make Love-Making Fun!..*11*

Getting to Baby: Communication Story 11

Go on Vacation!..*12*
Consider Acupuncture...*13*
Manage Your Time and Energy..*13*

**CHAPTER 2 Preparing Yourself and Your Partner Emotionally for the
Ups and Downs of the Journey** 15

Returning Blood Stain...*15*

How to Deal with a Miscarriage—
    From Someone Who Has Lived It..*16*
Create a Response In Advance..*17*
It May Be Time for a Diagnosis *18*
How to Stay Centered When Everyone Else is Pregnant *18*

Getting to Baby: Staying Centered Story **18**

Letting Go and Knowing When
    to Consider Alternative Methods...*23*
Research Alternatives...*24*
The Option No One Talks About..*25*
How to Deal with Overwhelm *25*

Getting to Baby: Adoption Option Story **26**

Where to Go From Here: Introducing Some Options.....................*27*

CHAPTER 3   Infertility Sucks! **29**

Why a Couple May Consider Fertility Treatments.........................*31*
Insemination—Artificial or Otherwise — What Is Artificial
    Insemination and why should you consider it? *33*
The Potential Risks of Informal Insemination...............................*35*
Receiving Help from a Willing Male That You Know.....................*36*

Getting to Baby: Artificial Insemination Story **36**

Put it All in Writing: The Importance of a Contract *37*
Getting the Sperm You Want...*37*
Deciding How Much Sperm to Buy...*39*
Artificial Insemination (AI): In Vitro Insemination (IVF) and
    Intrauterine Insemination (IUI) *40*
Intrauterine Insemination (IUI) *41*
Physician Assisted vs. Doing it at Home?......................................*41*
Tips for Artificial Insemination *42*
More on Costs, Insurance Coverage and Add-Ons........................*43*
In Vitro Fertilization (IVF)..*45*
Possible Hormonal Effects to Look Out For...................................*47*

Getting to Baby: In Vitro Fertilization Story............................. **48**

Multiple Medical Appointments: How to Prepare Yourself............*50*
Success with Fertility Assistance in 12 Months or Less.................*51*

Action Steps That Can Be Taken Now:
Finding the Right Doctor and Clinic...*52*
More Action Steps to Consider When Looking for the Right Fit.....*54*

CHAPTER 4   The Adoption Option **57**

Different Types of Adoption...*59*
Closed Adoptions...*59*
More on Closed Adoption...*61*
Semi-Open Adoption *61*
Open Adoption..*63*
The Importance of a Birth Mother Letter..................................*65*
Requirements for Most Adoption Options..................................*65*
Set a Strong Foundation and Network!......................................*66*
Hire a Marketing or Graphic Designer *66*
Consider Google AdWords *66*

Getting to Baby: Networking Story..................................... 67

Use Social Media and Viral Marketing.....................................*68*
Which Adoption Option is Best? *70*
Adopting Internationally *71*
Adoption Agencies and Facilitators..*73*
Important Questions to Ask When Choosing an Agency...............*74*

Getting to Baby: Adoption Story...**75**

What is an Adoption Facilitator?..*75*
Important Questions to ask
When Choosing an Adoption Facilitator...............................*76*

Getting to Baby: Adoption Facilitator Story **77**

Adoption Expenses *78*
Financial Relief: Our Own Experience......................................*79*
Adoption Scams and Warning Signs...*81*
Fun Facts about Adoption...*82*
Adoption Action Steps *84*
Adoption Checklist *84*

Getting to Baby: Adoption Story... 85

Getting to Baby: Adoption Story... 86

CHAPTER 5   Success with Surrogacy **87**

Getting to Baby: Surrogacy Story 88

Surrogacy Agencies *89*
"Want Ad" Websites *89*
Know the Different Types of Surrogacy *91*

Getting to Baby: Surrogacy Story 92

Seeking a Surrogate on Your Own *93*
Surrogates Look At You Too *94*
Why Do They Choose To Be a Surrogate? *95*
Matching with a Surrogate: What to Consider Before *96*
What to Include In a Surrogacy Contract *97*
Know Which States Allow Surrogacy *98*

Getting to Baby: Surrogacy Story 99

Decide on a Medical Plan *100*
Decide On a Birth Plan *102*

Getting to Baby: Surrogacy Story 102

Protecting the Surrogates Feelings *104*
Surrogacy Facts *107*
Surrogacy Checklist *108*
Action Steps That Can Be Taken Now *110*
Creating Your Family in 12 Months or Less *112*

CHAPTER 6   Expecting Multiples **117**

Difficult Decisions *118*
Twins *119*
Multiple Birth Facts *120*
Capturing the Experience through Pictures *122*
The Easter Bunny Brought
     Our Babies Home on Easter Sunday 2010 ....*127*
Second Parent Adoption Hearing *129*
Four Generations! *130*
ADORABLE!! *131*
First Christmas 2010 ....*132*

CHAPTER 7   Our Personal Stories Using Alternative Methods and Lessons We'd like to Pass On To You 133

Getting to Baby: Our Entire Story 133

Mr. Dreamy..*134*

Home Run! *135*

We Were High-Risk..*136*

To Have an Amniocentesis or Not? *137*

Something was Different This Time...................................*138*

What are Our Options? *139*

The Waiting Game...*140*

It's All in Pieces...*141*

Saying Goodbye *143*

Everything That Seems Certain Changes..........................*143*

Everyone Feels Loss Differently.......................................*145*

The Blessing of Support *147*

Meeting Sharon *150*

Watch the Scam Boards..*151*

What We Learned *152*

The Biggest Take-Away We Got...*153*

Time to Bring in the Adoption Facilitator........................*153*

Why We Felt She Was Reputable *154*

Texas and the Aries Baby *154*

Why it Sounded Like a Match...*155*

What Happened..*155*

The Day of the Birth...*156*

The Phone Call...*156*

The Aftermath..*157*

A Time for Questions..*158*

Self-Reflection and Transparent Beliefs *160*

The Big Ah-Ha! *160*

Another Light Bulb...*161*

What do you think about Surrogacy? *162*

Getting to Baby Surrogacy Story: Victory! 162

Research and Responses *163*

Brittany..*164*

The Match...*165*

Moving Closer..*166*

Setting Parameters *167*
The Process *168*
Everything Doesn't Always Go As Planned *169*
The Benefits of Us Planning Ahead *170*
Cervical Cerclage *171*
Decision Time *172*
Not Again! *173*
The Fun Doctor *173*
The Waiting Game *175*
Moment of Truth *175*
Back to Brittany *176*
Her Body, Our Children *176*
Baby Showers *177*
The Big Day: Countdown to Baby *179*
Ready for Their Close-Ups: Christopher and Katherine *180*
Post-Birth *182*
Rush-Hour in Atlanta *182*
The House and Brittany *183*
A Fork in the Road *184*
Keeping in Touch *184*
In Closing *185*

About the Authors **187**

BONUS OFFER **189**

Author's Note and Disclosure:

We are Victoria and Jennifer Collier. If you are reading this, you want to create a family or have a loved one who does. When we set out to create our family, we followed the "typical" roadmap many couples take on their journey. It was a long and at times heartbreaking journey for us. We started with fertility, specifically In-Vitro Fertilization (IVF). We suffered a miscarriage, two subsequent negative pregnancy test results, and broken hearts. What's next on the roadmap? Adoption. So, we began the adoption process. We had some close calls and two failed adoptions, once again breaking our hearts. We began to feel this was the end of the road for us. Then we learned of surrogacy. This proved to be the fast-lane getting us to baby. We want to share our experience with you to help you find your fast-lane. Knowledge is power and having the knowledge before you begin can help you streamline your process, making your journey one of triumph rather than heartbreak.

Disclosure: The information in this book is not intended to substitute for medical or legal expertise and advice. We encourage you to discuss any decisions about treatment or care with your healthcare provider and legal issues with an attorney. The attorney you use should be experienced and knowledgeable about assisted reproductive technology, adoption, or surrogacy. To find such attorney, search attorneys who are members of the American Academy of Adoption Attorneys (AAAA) and the American Academy of Reproductive Technology Attorneys (AARTA).

Baby's Face

Baby's face, a peaceful place
Full of wonder, no adult issues to ponder
Everything exciting and new
I believe I would like one, or perhaps even two

We know how important having a family is to you and wherever you find yourself in the process, we want you to know that it IS possible, because we have lived it ourselves. There was nothing more exciting than looking into our beautiful twin babies' eyes and knowing that against so many odds, we were finally parents! And you can be too. The important thing to know is that you CAN create your family and you are NOT alone.

In this book, we'll be sharing our personal journey with you and giving you the insider perspective on everything from how to prepare yourself to different alternative methods and what to ask when making those important choices. Just by the fact that you are picking up the book tells us that you are someone who is committed and dedicated to learning as much as possible about this transformation called parenthood. Our intention is to both inform and offer suggestions that we wish someone would have shared with us when we started and we encourage you to connect with us after reading the book through www.GettingtoBaby.com. Now let's get you to baby!

CHAPTER 1

Preparing to Create Your Family Now

"It is not good enough for things to be planned, they still have to be done; for the intention to become a reality, energy has to be launched into operation." —Walt Kelly

Where is Your Mind?

How long have you been trying to get pregnant?

What methods have been used?

Have you been trying the same method or have you experimented with alternative methods?

I remember feeling overwhelmed when someone would ask me those questions when Jennifer and I first started sharing with people that we wanted to be parents. If someone has asked you those questions recently, or perhaps you have asked them of yourself, realize that the question behind the question lies in your mind. What is *your* driving force behind wanting to have a child?

Your mindset directly impacts the methods you choose to try to get pregnant or have a child. It also affects how well you cope with stress. If you are going for a traditional pregnancy with a spouse there are things you have to look at. Have you been doing the same activities week after week? Have you tried spicing it up, or have you seen a fertility specialist?

What options have you looked at? Do you have other children? Having other children may have positive effects on trying to get pregnant again, but it may also trigger some negative thoughts such as: *I've done this before, why can't I do it now?*

Not having children can affect your mindset of having a child because you probably are thinking things like: *Everybody else has children, why can't I? I just want one child, why can't I have one child?* Whether or not you already have children can change your mindset, which can have an effect on your pregnancy or ability to have children.

Could your age be a factor? Many people are waiting longer to have children, waiting until their careers are under way. People are waiting longer to get married which means that they're generally older when they start the process of having children. If you're a non-traditional or same sex couple, then you have different issues to consider when thinking about creating your family.

There are also societal assumptions. For the most part, if you are in your early 20s, you're not being pressured to have children yet. As you age, people start asking you if you are ever going to have children. Those kinds of pressures can add stress and make you choose to do things that you otherwise may not have done.

For gay couples, the question is- *How* you are you going to get pregnant? For example, many people assume for example that with a lesbian couple, one of the women can just have the child as if it's as easy as going to the supermarket. People assume that a gay man or gay couple is going to adopt a child.

It's easier to know and deal with the assumptions that are out there. That way you can understand how you're going to either comply with those assumptions, stray from those, and be able to answer for yourself what your comfort level is.

The bottom line is that you have to answer for yourself why you want to have a baby right now, not years ago, not in two years from now, but right now. What is the driving force behind having a child and creating a family today? Doing that sort of self-reflection can help you put priorities in place, clear the clutter that may prevent you from going forward and having children and focus your life so that if in fact, you do want that child today, right now, that you can put in motion what's necessary to create that.

Getting On The Same Page: The Importance of Communication, Care-Giving and Setting a Budget

Regardless of age, lifestyle or health, there are many things to consider when you're getting pregnant or having a baby any other way. It's not just a matter of saying we want a baby, and we can make it work flawlessly. You've got people, conditions and finances to consider.

In order to create your beautiful family right now and alleviate potential stress and strain throughout that process, it is essential that couples be at or near the same place in their minds and hearts. There are things that can be done to be sure you and your partner are on the same page, but communication is the number one key factor.

Note: If you are not in a relationship, these are all still relevant topics to discuss with your support system and yourself before embarking on this journey.

Having discussions and talking is paramount. And those talks should not always center around wanting a baby, because that's what the discussion generally is about. I want a baby. Why? Well, I just do. It needs to be why do we *both* want this right now? This is not as a couple, but individually, where you can share your own thoughts, feelings, fears and hopes. Then you can look at it as a couple to see if each of your reasons mesh together, which is important.

Do career issues work out? For example, have you discussed realistically if both parents will work? Will one parent stay at home? Will there need to be childcare? Who will be the primary caregiver? That doesn't necessarily mean that someone is going to stay home with the child, but there are roles that become self-defined as a relationship develops and one of those roles is being the primary caregiver for the children. Who is that going to be? Especially, with heterosexual couples, society defines those roles to which people play along very nicely with the female as the primary caregiver and the male as the financial provider.

With lesbian and gay families, society doesn't have any preconceived expectations about who is going to be the primary caregiver. Thus, those are issues that should be discussed in advance. That way, it's more natural after the child becomes part of the family.

Today men are a lot more involved as parents than they were historically. Men will take their children to swimming lessons, extra curricular activities and show up at school. Having a discussion of roles and involvement beforehand is very important because we all create our own expectations in our minds as to how things are going to play out. One of the biggest issues with relationships is that we build up expectations in our mind and then the situations don't happen the way we thought they would or should, then we get upset and frustrated. Usually this is because we failed to communicate our expectation. This is about starting the discussions to communicate our expectations and one of those expectations is the involvement of the parents and what will that be.

Set a Budget

Another important issue when you begin to plan a family is setting a budget. When you can get pregnant without the use of fertility treatments, adoption or surrogacy, becoming pregnant is very inexpensive. If you have issues that lead you down the fertility, adoption or surrogacy route, it can become very expensive, very fast. You must understand what your financial means are and set a budget so that you don't go over that.

Let's say you had good intentions of setting a budget but at some point you get so emotionally involved in wanting a child and creating your family that the budget is thrown out the window. Worse, if you didn't create a budget, then you don't even have a clue of how much you've been spending because you haven't been keeping track. You can find yourself upside down financially very quickly.

One of the important things to remember is that once you have that child, you still need money to raise the child, so you don't want to spend all of it on the process. Sitting down and creating a budget is important. This may be the very first time that a couple has sat down together and reviewed the finances and determined a plan together.

This is a joint decision. It affects both people equally, not just personally but also financially, so from the beginning, both people need to understand what their capabilities are and then support each other with that. And when everything is put out on the table, you will be more than ready to conquer the more difficult questions that may present themselves.

It's Not a Perfect World
•••••••••••••••••••••••••••

Another discussion that you may need to have is, What if the child is born with disabilities? When you think about getting pregnant or adopting a child or creating a child in other ways, of course, it's normal to believe that it's going to be the most perfect world and that having a baby will make all of your dreams come true. Sometimes babies are born with physical or mental disabilities. Knowing how you would react to that is important. If age is a factor as to why you're not getting pregnant, remember that age is a direct link to some abnormalities at birth, such as Down syndrome.

You can't bury your head in the sand and hope that it's not going to happen to you. And, when people are looking into adoption, one of the questions asked when you are filling out a profile as to what type of child you are willing to adopt is: *Are you willing to accept a child with mild, moderate or severe disabilities?* That is an important question that you might not have considered.

When creating the plan to have a child and a family, what is commonly forgotten is a back up plan. What if the pregnancy is not successful? Think about what you would do, what options you would take, what research you would conduct if your pregnancy were not successful.

For heterosexual families, much of this thinking is not done in advance because people just love each other, they get pregnant and they have babies. It's not until there is a problem that they start looking into these concerns. Lesbian and gay couples, cannot accidentally have children, thus, they must plan out their course of action before they can have a child.

These are issues that everyone should think about even before they start to create their family. Dealing with those uncomfortable, difficult questions early on can potentially benefit you down the road. And you will be glad you addressed them up front!

Discussing Alternatives With Each Other
• •

Not everyone is comfortable with adoption, surrogacy, or fertility treatment and the hormones that a person must take during that process. When we were going through the fertility process, we knew of many couples that had tried artificial insemination, 6, 10 or 15 times. Every time you have an unsuccessful procedure, it feels like such a loss. You go through the five stages of loss and grief: denial, anger, bargaining, depression, and acceptance. To go through that process over and over can certainly have an effect on you in many different ways. From the beginning, set a time frame of when to consider your alternatives.

Have a Support Team
· · · · · · · · · · · · · · · · · · · ·

Your support system can be family, friends, your partner or spouse and may very well include all of those. It can be people you know very well, who know you very well, or it can even be people you haven't talked to in a long time.

For example, my support system is my partner Jennifer, and I have one very good friend who's a support person who I can talk to about anything. She doesn't have her own children and has never wanted children, so it doesn't have to be someone who's gone through what you have gone through. You'll be grateful to have the support system when you have big news to share!

Getting to Baby: Communication Story

"Do you tell your families that you're pregnant? Or, should you wait 12 weeks because that is the critical stage?" We both asked ourselves this question when we first found out that we were expecting a child via In-vitro fertilization, which we'll talk about later in the book. I'm the kind of person who can't wait. I want immediate results, and I want to share with the world my immediate results – certainly those so rewarding as being pregnant. Jennifer, on the other hand, is much more self-disciplined. To get back on the same page, we had a compromise that allowed me to tell strangers, but I couldn't tell people closest to us. I told the person who was caring for my dog and people that we weren't super close to. It worked out for both of us because it was important for me to respect Jennifer's view and for her to respect the fact that I couldn't keep my mouth shut.

We lost our child after a medical procedure at 17 weeks which was after the 12 weeks safe harbor period. So even if I had waited 12 weeks to tell everyone, the result would have been the same—everyone would have known. The difference is that they, our support system, were with us along the way. When things did not turn out the way we had hoped at any point throughout our process, they were still with us. If I had to have carried that burden by myself, I'm not sure I personally could have been able to do it. Have discussions with your support system, with the people you choose to rely on emotionally through your process, whether the news is positive or negative.

Also, remember to discuss the boundaries between you and your support system.

- How often can you whine to them when things are difficult?
- Do you want them to give you advice or do you just want them to listen to you and support and provide a lending ear or shoulder?
- Do you want them to just let you cry?
- Do you want them to tell you it's going to be okay?
- Would that be the worst thing they can say to you?

Everybody needs something different. We all have our own ideas as to what we expect from others, but unless you convey that to your support system, they might not know what to do or say. Yet, they want to support you in the way that you need. It's much easier to share that with them *before* you're in a struggle than it is *while* you're in a struggle because then you get frustrated. You may say, "Oh, you just don't understand me," and leave. This leads to total frustration for both sides.

This communication is especially important between spouses and partners. It doesn't matter if you are different or the same gender, you're not always going to understand each other. In summary, your language may not be the same as someone else's, so be clear on what your needs are so your support team can do their job!

Finding Support Through Social Media: Facebook

Surprisingly, throughout the adoption process, I found a lot of support on Facebook from friends I went to high school with. I'm 40 years old and while I enjoy the Internet, I'm not much into social networking. Jennifer and I both feel the same way. Until we went through the adoption process, we would never have said our own names in the same sentence as Facebook, other than: "Victoria will not do Facebook."

Think outside the box. Don't just think about who is there every day for you. Think about who could be right for you in that moment. We got a Facebook page, and we started reaching out to people who we were in high school with. Two of them became my biggest support system when going through the adoption process, which I could have never, ever predicted in advance.

Different Strokes for Different Folks:
The Importance of a Positive Attitude and Self-Care

Having a positive attitude and taking care of yourself are paramount to getting you ready for your baby. Here are a few tips for both couples and individuals to keep in mind.

Make Love-Making Fun!

As a society we all tend to multi-task to get so much done that we continue to add stress to our bodies. Seeing lovemaking as fun instead of a chore is essential.

Getting to Baby: Communication Story

I had a heterosexual lawyer friend and he and his wife were trying to get pregnant the same time Jennifer and I were trying to get pregnant. We'd have telephone conferences, and he would have to get off the phone because that's when his wife needed him at home, and we'd have to reschedule the teleconference. I found it to be extremely funny and he didn't. Over time, he dreaded going home in the middle of the day or at any time because he felt like he became a tool and not a participant in a relationship with the same goal.

Make it fun. Do the things you did in the first year of your marriage or partnership. Do it in the places that you wouldn't normally do it. Do it at times you wouldn't normally do it. Become that first year relationship again, if for no other purpose than to relax, have fun and create a baby.

Regardless of your lifestyle, you have to keep the making love aspect in tact. It will feel better, especially when you do achieve the success that you're looking for because you'll remember that "moment of conception" and instead of "that situation." It will be the, "Oh, it was up against the wall when we snuck out of the party early…" It would be a moment to look back on with fondness.

Go on Vacation!

This takes us to another point—go on vacation. You may be thinking that now is not a good time for you to take time off work because you're trying to save vacation leave for when you have the baby, not to mention saving money for when the baby arrives. Vacation doesn't have to be a weeklong adventure. You can go on weekend trips. The whole idea is to relax, return to who you are and enjoy yourself so that you can create your baby.

Think creatively. Vacation can even be in your own city. Maybe it's at the nice hotel down the street that you would never go to on a regular occasion, but this just might be that special occasion.

Consider Acupuncture

In our process, we also used acupuncture, which is not a Western medical procedure. Acupuncture can help your body relax. When your body is relaxed, your blood is flowing the way it should and pregnancy can occur more easily.

Manage Your Time and Energy

I can tell you that as a lawyer who owns her own law practice, I was working no less than 70 hours a week before having children. It became clear that I had "stuff" cluttering my life because I didn't have the children filling my life or my time. Now that I do have children, out of necessity I've had to de-clutter the other, less important time-sucking activities.

I am now down to 50 hours a week. I never thought that I could still be successful and cut 20 hours out of my work schedule. But I am, and even more successful! If I had worried myself the whole time trying to have a child knowing I could no longer work 70 hours a week and wondering how I would get everything done, I would have stressed myself out. There were so many things I could have worried about such as: *How am I going to be able to serve my clients the way they've come to expect?, How will they react to me changing the way I've always done it in the past?, What if they decide to leave and go somewhere else? Will I be able to spend enough time with my children?*

If I were so focused on that that I didn't create an alternate plan for this drastic change, my body would have been so tense that it may never have allowed a child to come into my life. Instead, with foresight and planning, I was able to hire more employees/support staff and it was truly a win-win situation.

With your life as busy as it is, it is essential to schedule in "time to plan." Take the time off from work to interview physicians or adoption agencies that can help. Do what's necessary. There are no accidents in the way we get pregnant so everything is a deliberate choice. Make time in your schedule to see the appropriate doctors and do your research. Ultimately clear your life of clutter and try to de-stress. Sit down and think about what currently takes the majority of your attention and time. Are these things necessary in your life or are you just letting them fill your life because you don't have anything filling that spot for the moment?

Look in advance where the time that you are going to create is going to come from. You'll have to make time for the children. Take a look around. See what you can create in your life that promotes peace, calmness and less stress. When you can identify that and make an alternate plan for those things, you'll be ahead of the game.

To share with you why I know this is possible, I used to work 70 hours or more per week. Now, I am able to wake my children each day at 6:00 a.m., feed them, and play with them until 8:15 a.m.. Then, I take off from work from 11:15 a.m. through 12:30 p.m. each day to attend swimming lessons. Lastly, I am home each night by 6:00 p.m. to play, give baths, feed, and tuck them into bed each night by 7:45 p.m.. Do you think our lives have changed? You bet! But we planned for it.

CHAPTER 2

"Preparing Yourself and Your Partner Emotionally for the Ups and Downs of the Journey."

RETURNING BLOOD STAIN

A desperate lesbian sings of a new life
Shared between herself and her beautiful wife
To see bright eyes and a smiling face
To dress him in sneakers or her in lace
Try after try, we commit a sin
For this new love, we'd do it again
Yet time after time we shade our pain
Of month after month that returning blood stain

Before we had the joy of our twins, there were a number of challenging experiences that we both went through. And wherever you are on your journey, we intend to help you feel as supported as possible throughout the inevitable ups and downs. The challenging times can make the victorious ones seem that much sweeter.

I wrote that poem in 1990, and even to this day, I well up in tears every time I read it because for a couple that really wants to create their family, there is both an emotional and physical reaction. When you're trying to get pregnant, every single month your period is a reminder that you are not. Each month I would think to myself: *That damned period again. Here it is!* When you're young and carefree, you want to see that period every month but when you're trying so hard to get pregnant, it becomes your worst enemy.

For lesbian couples, it depends on who's trying to get pregnant as far as how you might react. With a heterosexual relationship, men may have a more positive attitude because they know they have more sperm and will try again, unless they have been diagnosed with a low sperm count. When pregnancy doesn't happen quickly, the first reaction people have is to try harder to get pregnant. You might get frustrated, mad at each other and start getting short and snippy with each other. Then you don't understand what's wrong with the relationship. You may just be trying too hard.

How to Deal with a Miscarriage—
From Someone Who Has Lived It

Sometimes you get pregnant, sometimes you don't. Having a miscarriage is a totally different situation. Having a miscarriage is difficult for everyone involved. It's a grief emotion, and it can affect couples trying to create a family very differently.

For a female, you go to the restroom and you have a period-like situation except that it's different and you know it's different because it's not a bloodstain, it's a much larger indicator. The woman has to live through that experience. You want to grab into the toilet and bring your baby back. You want to put it back inside. You're generally alone because you go to the restroom by yourself. That walk from the restroom to wherever you are going next is a long one because you have to share that information with your husband or partner. Those words aren't easy to get out of your mouth.

The partner or husband wants to be as supportive as possible, but they don't feel what you're going through and couldn't possibly. They don't know the right thing to say, as if there is a right thing to say. That alone can cause strain in the relationship.

Unfortunately, some people have multiple miscarriages before they're successful in creating their family. While some people could get through it alone, I believe that no one should have to and it is so much better if you have a support system. Part of that support system can and should be your partner.

Some of that miscarriage emotion is that you've spent all of these months so thrilled to be pregnant. Whether you've told people or not, you're excited about it. Assuming the 12 weeks were up, you've told the whole world that you're pregnant. The loss creates not just the loss of expecting but you are also embarrassed because you've told everyone. You think that you're broken as a person, so you feel shame and failure. All of these emotions are going on when you have a miscarriage, and they must be dealt with. Just trying to get pregnant again does not erase the loss. That is one of the reasons why these potential issues should be discussed in the beginning and that you have a plan to help you get through a situation if it in fact does happen.

Create a Response In Advance

I recommend that people create a response in advance. As horrible as it is, you have to think about that if you have a miscarriage, if you've told the whole world you're pregnant, you have to say something. By writing it out ahead of time, you avoid being caught off guard when someone asks how your pregnancy is going. My canned response became: "It hasn't developed the way we wanted it to." People knew that wasn't a positive response and that I'd share more information if I chose to. They got the message not to ask me any more questions. This is a personal thing between partners that they each must individually decide for themselves and then discuss as partners how to present it when together. There is no one response. But having one that's been practiced and rehearsed so that it comes out more naturally can help you feel more prepared and ease the burden of grief.

It May Be Time for a Diagnosis

If you've been trying and trying, then maybe it's time to get a diagnosis. Determine why you are not getting pregnant. *Is there a low sperm count? Are you making love too often? Is there an egg issue?* When Jennifer and I went through the fertility process, I found out that I had a low egg count and the eggs that I produce are weak in nature. It didn't mean that I couldn't get pregnant, but it meant that success would be more difficult. It also meant that with weak eggs, a baby could have disabilities. Get a diagnosis. Have some tests done and then make decisions whether to keep trying or to look into a different process.

How to Stay Centered When Everyone Else is Pregnant

It seems like when you are trying to get pregnant, everyone else you know and see is having a baby. It's similar to when you buy a new car. You drive it off the lot and you see 20 other cars drive by you with the exact same model and color. It's the same with pregnancy. What you focus on is what you see more of and what you are surrounded by. When you're focused so much on getting to baby, all you can see, everywhere you look, is pregnant women and babies.

Getting to Baby: Staying Centered Story

We had been on our journey for at least four years and we were still trying to create our family. I was at the Post Office, standing in line waiting to mail a package. There was a lady standing in front of me who looked younger than I was and didn't look financially stable. She was definitely pregnant, like at any moment she could have this child.

I stood there for a good 10 minutes and thinking in my head the entire time: *How can I start up a conversation to ask her if she wants that child? Can I have your child? Can I adopt your child, because I know I could provide for this child?* She put her package on top of the counter, and I saw that it was going overseas so I just created a conversation out of that. "Are you from England?" I asked. She told me she was.

What I was trying to discover was if she was married because she wasn't wearing a wedding ring. It was probably because she was swelling. Ultimately, the story led to the fact that she was in fact married and this was her second child and she was very much looking forward to it. The point was that as happy as I was for her, I realized how much I wanted to be pregnant too.

Some tips that you can use to stay centered are:

1. It is important to try to control your emotions.

Otherwise, you will be crying every time you see a baby or pregnant lady. You find yourself in situations where you do things that you wouldn't otherwise do just because you see babies all around you. You become very social. There are other situations that come up that almost rip your heart out. For example, in my law practice, I serve elderly clients. I had a client who had a granddaughter. She was 18 years old and got pregnant by her boyfriend. They were raising this child together.

They were in a car without the baby in a car seat, and they had a major accident. Both parents died and another child, not theirs, was in the car and died. Their baby flew out of the window, and by God's grace alone, it survived the accident. Now, the infant is living with people who are not its parents. I wanted to scream at how irresponsible I felt that was and how much better I would be as a mom, but instead I had to keep my emotions in check.

2. You may experience anger and that is okay.

To hear of a situation like I described above after trying to have our child for so long was heart wrenching. Some of my thoughts were: *Here we're doing everything we can to have a baby and seeing people like this who aren't taking proper care of their beautiful baby makes me so mad! She might as well have thrown the baby out from the car herself.*

Understand that these situations are out of your control but you can control your reaction to them.

3. You have to create positive outlets and other support groups.

While you can say these things to try to find some humor in your process, it is downright frustrating and it can eat at you if you let it. You have to find outlets so that you're not always focusing on the negative. Otherwise, that's all you'll see in your life. That's another reason why having a support system is so important. They can see things more objectively than you.

You need to put yourself in groups of like-minded people. While, your support system doesn't have to include someone who has been through everything that you've been through, once in a while, it is nice to talk with somebody who has been through what you've been through. On some level, they'll understand how you feel, understand what you've gone through, and help push you through some "stuck" moments.

For example, in my situation, as a lesbian I would not be as comfortable going to a support group of strictly heterosexual women that could not get pregnant because their issues may be different. They might look at me differently, or at least, that may be my perception. I would look for a support group of other lesbian couples that were trying to get pregnant through artificial insemination (AI) or In Vitro Fertilization (IVF).

There are support groups for men who have low sperm count or who have other fertility issues that are affecting a pregnancy. While you might not think of men as having emotions as much as women, the man's experience also affects his ability to be part of that relationship and to support his spouse or partner going forward on the path to create a child.

4. Celebrate the successes of others

After we lost our child, a woman Jennifer worked with was pregnant at the same time we were pregnant. Her baby was due two days after our baby. She had her child, and she was so afraid to show excitement in front of us that she just didn't. We felt very touched that she was concerned about our feelings, but we had already gotten our emotions under control and knew how to deal with that situation. It's just a matter of finding those positive outlets to do that. You can be sad for your own situation, but still be happy for others.

5. Have Faith

Having faith means having the belief in something you cannot see or prove. At your core, have faith that this will happen for you. Ultimately, it is about believing that your child will come when he/she is supposed to. Jennifer and I had to believe. When we got pregnant and lost that child, one of the faiths that we returned to is that we had always wanted twins. Jennifer is a twin. We couldn't decide if we wanted a girl or a boy so we deliberately decided we wanted both and that we only wanted to go through the process once, so twins was our answer. When we lost our first child, a girl, it was absolutely devastating to us. But, our faith kept us strong and we truly believed that our girl was not ready to be with us until her brother could be with us too. Currently we have twins: a girl and a boy. We feel that our children came to us when they were ready to do so. And seeing their faces everyday is a constant reminder for us to have faith.

6. Seek Out Professional Counseling

Of course, professional counseling is an option. It is something that should be considered if someone feels that their emotions are affecting their daily activities. You would want to consider professional help if you are not able to do the same things that you normally enjoy doing or were doing because of emotions that are linked to not being able to get pregnant or create a family.

Recognize too, this is something that couples should talk about together. It's okay if only one person in the couple needs to go to professional counseling. It's okay if both of them do. It's also okay if they see the same counselor or if they want to see different counselors. It's certainly okay if neither of them needs counseling. In our situation, after we did the fertility treatment, got pregnant and then lost the child, I thought I was okay. My undergraduate degree is in psychology, so while I understood the benefits of counseling, I simply didn't think I needed it at the time.

I talked to all of my friends. I talked to Jennifer non-stop. We walk every night for exercise, and that was my time to really get out all of my feelings and emotions. Then I'd come into work and my staff knew what was going on. I realized that I was showing up to work and just going through the motions. I had a practice that I had built from nothing to making a lot of money and helping a lot of families. I just didn't care about those families anymore the way I had before. I could not have cared less if their file sat on my desk for another day, week or a month.

I remember one day where I was sitting at my desk feeling numb. I wasn't going through what I thought was a typical depression with being irritable, crying and sleeping all the time. All I knew was that I just didn't care about anything. That is when I decided I wanted and needed to care. I knew I needed someone to help me because while my support system was good, I needed more, so I went to counseling.

What I didn't understand was, *Why didn't Jennifer feel she needed counseling?* She wasn't nearly as verbose as I was. She didn't explain all of her deepest feelings to me all the time or to anybody. *Why was I the only one?* I realized that it didn't really matter. I needed that assistance; she did not. The Bottom Line: What really matters is that you seek the assistance you need to help yourself. We all cope with things differently, and that's okay.

Letting Go and Knowing When
to Consider Alternative Methods
• •

There are times when you have to move on and let go. The most important and sometimes most difficult part is knowing *when* to do that. Letting go of an attachment to one way of getting pregnant can be likened to letting go of a relationship that sometimes just isn't working out.

When you're with someone and you know the relationship is not going in the direction you want it to anymore and you've been together for quite a while, it's hard to let go. I have a couple of friends who have been together for over 10 years. They have been having difficulties for the last two years. They're still in the relationship. It's clear from all casual observers that the relationship is over, but they're just dragging it out, which is causing more pain to them.

While I am an absolute supporter of doing what is necessary and helpful to maintain a positive relationship for all parties involved, when it's over it's over. The same thing is true for getting pregnant and trying to get pregnant on your own. When you can't, you can't. It's at that point that you've got to consider alternative options.

Those alternative options can include a variety of things but before getting there, when you're trying to get pregnant set a time frame. In our case, we were going to work on getting pregnant for a year. If we were not pregnant 12 months from then, then we both agreed to seek professional advice, see if we could get a diagnosis, see if more aggressive fertility treatments were warranted or if we should just stop trying.

Let's briefly revisit the importance of setting a time frame. When you set that time frame, it is important to stick to it. Jennifer and I were 36 when we started our process of trying to get pregnant. We decided if we were not pregnant by the time we turned 38, we would start the adoption process. We knew that the adoption process could take years. We made a plan:

- At 36, we'll try to get pregnant.

- At 38, if we're not we will start the adoption process.

- At 40, if we are not in the process of actively adopting a child with a person we have matched with who has a child or is about to have a child, then we will stop all processes, and we will no longer try to have children. We will then decide how to creatively fulfill our lives together as a couple in a different way.

That is exactly what we did. We stuck with our plan but added a twist, which you'll read more about later.

Research Alternatives

Do research during that time frame of your process that you've put in place. This is the perfect time to do research on your alternatives because you don't need the alternative at that moment. It's the best emotional space for you to look for the alternative so that you can know that if you need a back up plan, it's there without the emotional charge of having to make the actual decisions. You've got the time to do the research now, so do it before your back up plan becomes your primary plan.

When you move on and let go and start looking at other options, you can feel very overwhelmed with all of the options available. *Do we get an infertility analysis? Do we go through fertility treatment*? There are so many different kinds of fertility treatments. There is artificial insemination, In Vitro Fertilization, egg and sperm donation, just to name a few. With each of those treatments, there are so many other things that need to be considered. Their cost is different, some take longer than others, and some require more medication and hormones than others. There are a lot of decisions that must be made for you to feel comfortable creating a child in that way. It can be very overwhelming. When researching alternatives, go to www.GettingtoBaby.com for a list of questions you should ask yourself and ask medical professionals.

You might think, "We can't get pregnant, so let's just adopt." Surrogacy is an option that is often overlooked. This is how we became successful at creating our family. It's almost like a secret option, but it's certainly a rising option.

The Option No One Talks About

An option that no one talks about but some couples ultimately do is the decision to live without children. As mentioned, Jennifer and I decided that at the age of 40, if we did not have a child, we would move forward and create our life differently, positively and without children.

The way you look at it can have an effect on whether you're going to get pregnant along the way or create that adoption or surrogate situation because it affects your mood and outlook. There's a difference between *making the decision that it's okay to move forward without children* and *resigning yourself to not having them*. Decide that it's okay to have a different life at that point and what your life is going to be. Don't just let it happen. Your mindset can help you through your process.

How to Deal with Overwhelm

It can be overwhelming when looking at the options, especially if you go on the Internet. For example, with adoption, there are thousands of different sites that all want your attention. Talk it to death between you and your partner. Talk about all the options. *What are the pros and cons of this or that option? How do you feel when you hear the word fertility or adoption?* We all have our own visceral emotional feelings that are attached to certain things and knowing what yours are can be helpful.

Getting to Baby: Adoption Option Story

I have some friends, a husband and a wife, that were having some fertility issues and weren't getting pregnant. They were getting older which their physician felt was one of their contributing factors to not getting pregnant. They started discussing adoption.

The woman was all for adoption. In fact, she was okay without even trying to get pregnant because she didn't want to put her body through what a body goes through when it's pregnant. Thank goodness they had good communication, because the husband, on the other hand didn't feel it was a good option for them. He jokingly said something that he was serious about. He felt he needed the genetic bond between himself and his child. He said: "When that child makes me angry, I think I'll be able to restrain myself much easier if there is a genetic bond."

Anyone who is or who has adopted and is reading this book will likely get very upset with that statement because they know the bond is the same. Your child is your child regardless of how it came to you. I feel that way, but he did not. It was important for him to have shared that with his wife so she would know that adoption might never be an option for them.

When you've decided as a couple what your plan is going to be, make a commitment to that plan. Don't try to continue down two paths at once. That is like having a wife and a mistress or a husband and an affair on the side. Your attention is in two different areas and therefore you can't be wholly 100% successful in one area if you're dividing your attention to something else. Be committed to it and work on that new plan together.

Where to Go From Here: Introducing Some Options

The majority of people will go through fertility treatments. At some point in the future, like in our situation, as a lesbian couple, we could have adopted a child. Many lesbian couples do that without even going through fertility. However, for us, we would have always wondered if we could have had our own child.

Fertility treatments may be the first course you have to go through and hopefully the last, but if not, then it's a necessary step in the process. If it doesn't happen through fertility, then you go through the emotional thought of just wanting a child. It doesn't have to be our own child. We just want a child. I think society has played into the fact of what we think of adoption. *I can't have a child, so I'll adopt a child.* There are billboards everywhere for adoption. There are movies and television specials on adoption. Everybody knows somebody who has a friend that's adopted or someone in his or her family is adopted.

Of course, we love them just like we would love our own naturally born child. Adoption seems like the natural next step, but it isn't for everyone. It certainly wasn't for my friend who was afraid of hurting the child. There are other options to consider.

Another option is surrogacy. What is surrogacy? It's not something that you may have heard a lot about. It's becoming much more known because of the celebrities who are using surrogates to create their families. Using a surrogate, at its core, is creating a child with a third person, a woman, who is willing to carry that child to term for you.

Those are some of the options to get to baby. At the end of the day, you want a child. And we believe you can. Let's look at some of these alternative methods up close and personal to help you make that happen.

CHAPTER 3
Infertility Sucks!

**Exploring Alternative Methods: What They Are,
How they Work and How to Pick What Works for YOU!**

"Courage doesn't always roar. Sometimes courage is the quiet voice at the end of the day saying, I will try again tomorrow."
— *Mary Anne Radmacher*

Congratulations! You've done your homework, you know all the answers to questions that come up in the pre-planning and you and your partner are finally on the same page about everything and are both fully prepped on some of the ways you can emotionally support each other.

There's just one small thing. You are still having trouble getting pregnant. Whether you are in a heterosexual or homosexual relationship, let's discuss some alternative methods that you can consider. But before we dive in, we need to address the issue of infertility.

We know that infertility can be very frustrating but the good news it that there are many effective ways to cope with it. First let's look at the most common causes.

1. Age

Age is a factor that stands out as one of the main causes of infertility. People are waiting longer to get married; they are putting their careers first and babies second. Then there is the 50% divorce rate of people who marry. They're having children with their second and third marriages, so they're older when having children and adding to the family.

There are other causes too.

2. Abortions and Medical Procedures

Prior abortions and medical procedures can have a bearing on having children in the future due to scarring. Also, difficulty with an earlier pregnancy has some effects on future pregnancy.

A family member of mine had a successful pregnancy with her first child, but the child's head was extremely large so they had to use forceps to pull him out. Because his head was so large, the birthing process caused her fallopian tubes to be shorter than average, making subsequent pregnancies more difficult.

She tried to get pregnant multiple times since he was born. Her son is 16 years old now. While she has gotten pregnant, the pregnancies were not sustainable because of the lengths of her tubes. Prior difficult pregnancies or deliveries can create issues later.

3. Stress

The everyday stress that we talked about earlier also plays a part. If you're not at peace in your body, you're not at peace in what's going on around you and in your world. That stress can create a block from success in getting pregnant.

With heterosexual couples, assuming everything is working well, you don't have a lot of stress, and you're of good fertility age, by and large you will get pregnant. Same gender couples will never get pregnant that way. If it's a lesbian couple, they're missing the sperm. If it's a gay male couple, they're missing the egg.

There are certainly more causes than those but those are the common causes that a casual observer, a non-expert, can look across our society and see what's contributing to infertility.

Why a Couple May Consider Fertility Treatments

From a couple's perspective, they want their own child. If you can't get pregnant on your own, or get a diagnosis, then having a fertility treatment plan can help move you forward in the process. People want their own children because they want someone who's of their own flesh and blood. They want someone who looks and acts like them, who can carry on the family traditions through name and genetics.

They're also afraid of potentially not bonding with the child. While there are tons of wonderful adoption success stories with regard to children and their parents bonding, there are also some stories where the child and the parents did not bond. That obviously can happen with your own genetic children, too, but the perception is what leads them to do fertility treatment assistance and that perception, whether it's based on reality, is how decisions are made.

That takes me back to my friend who expressed to his wife that adoption would not be an option for him because he was afraid of the lack of bonding that could occur. Fertility treatments, and there are so many different variations of that, can seem the natural way to go. Fertility treatments are generally quicker and less expensive than adoption, which can take years.

Let's take artificial insemination (AI) for example. We will assume that the couple has a sperm issue, so they need sperm. You can buy a vial of sperm for just over $100 and that can be inseminated into the woman either by the husband, partner or by the physician. Assuming that's successful, you've spent very little money. Compared to adoption that can be anywhere from $10,000 to $50,000, AI can be much less expensive, quicker, and more natural option for some. However, it is not legal in some states for anyone other than a licensed physician to administer or perform artificial insemination. For example, in Georgia, it is a felony punishable by up to five years in prison. Do your research and consider consulting a lawyer in your area beforehand just to be safe.

For me, I would always wonder could I have had my own child if I didn't at least try this. *If I had just gone through that process, could I have had my own child, genetically?*

There is a lot of success with fertility treatments. There are OBGYN's and fertility specialists all over the world offering these services. Even when fertility assistance is not successful, I feel that it is a necessary evil that we all do before we explore other options. It's that one chance at having a child that came from us.

When we were going through our getting to baby process, we did all of the things I'm talking about so far. We communicated constantly and set our timeline, including how many times to do fertility treatments.

Jennifer and I decided that we would only do the fertility treatment two times, based on the hormones that we would have to inject into our bodies. The more you absorb, the more likely you could have side issues. Also the cost can become prohibitive.

The first time we did our IVF cycle, I produced very few eggs. Only one of them fertilized with the sperm, so we only had one egg that could be implanted for pregnancy. The second time we went through fertility, we had three eggs that fertilized. We did not want the high probability of having more than twins. The physician we were using, within her own ethics, would not even place more than two fertilized eggs in so we implanted both of those. We were not successful.

Then we had that one little egg out there that was fertilized, but we had set our limit at two tries. We've still got that one little egg, so what do we do? It comes down to the thought, *But what if I could have my own child?* We chose to go ahead and try to get pregnant with that one little egg. If we hadn't, it would always be on my mind. *What if that one little egg was the one?* Thanks to trying fertility treatments, that question was put to rest.

Insemination—Artificial or Otherwise
What Is Artificial Insemination and why should you consider it?

Artificial insemination (AI) is the process by which sperm is placed into the vaginal cavity. The sperm then swims through the fallopian tubes to find the eggs. Artificial insemination is used when the infertility issue is with the sperm. Either a male can't produce the sperm, hasn't got quality sperm, or there is no male in the equation. You have to have sperm for a pregnancy. Finding a willing participant is key.

There can be willing, unwilling and unknowing participants in the insemination process.

Let's talk specifically about a situation that lesbian couples who want to have a child can find themselves in and that is finding that willing participant. Lesbians, by and large don't make the same amount of income as a heterosexual couple where there is a male and a female either both working or let's stereotypically say the male is working. They don't make as much money as a gay couple where there are two men working. Still, in our society, men make more money than women and that is just a fact.

Lesbians may try to minimize the cost of creating children. It is not uncommon that lesbians will try to find a willing participant, such as a friend or stranger to get them pregnant. In order to do so, if having sex with a man is what that means, then some of them will do that in order to create their family. This is what I call "informal insemination."

If you're not inclined to want to have sex with a man because your orientation is towards women, then sometimes women use assistive aides such as alcohol to lower their inhibitions, making it more likely that they can go through that process. They'll have one-night stands until they are successful at their process.

I personally went through that process back in 1990. I had a partner for about a year when I was in the military. She and I wanted to have a child. I was 20 years old and she was 24. I've wanted to have a child ever since I was 19.

We were stationed together in Germany. We found a male friend who was 19. He was very cute and aesthetically pleasing. We approached him and told him what our desire was which was very risky given that we were both in the military. We were not supposed to be living that type of lifestyle.

That's the kind of thing you do when you want something so badly. You risk other factors of your life for it. It was worth it to us to have a child even if that meant we might get kicked out of the service if he were to share our secrets. He was a willing participant. We did what we needed to do to try to get pregnant which included having traditional intercourse with him. We tried that three times.

It was extremely painful emotionally and it created a wedge between my partner and me. Fortunately, I'm a huge believer in communication; the situation was something that she and I could communicate through. We were so interested in having children together that we took what I felt were desperate measures. Damn it, if that period didn't come every month thereafter.

That just gives you an idea of some of the things that can go on. It's not just lesbians that do that. If you're a child of the 80s, you might remember a song by Heart where she is singing about a situation where she and her husband could not get pregnant. She picked up a hitchhiker and had sex with him so that she could get pregnant and have a child. This is not isolated to one type of person who can't get pregnant. These things happen.

The Potential Risks of Informal Insemination
●●●

1. STD's

There are certainly some risks, one being the relationship between the partners, social issues such as sexually transmitted diseases, and you do not know the medical history of that person if he is a stranger. You don't know the family history of the person or if there are any mental health issues and things like that. Moreover, even when using the sperm of a known donor, it is essential to have the sperm clinically tested for diseases to include **human immunodeficiency virus (HIV)** which can cause acquired immunodeficiency syndrome (AIDS).

2. Legalities and Paternity Issues

Insemination can also create legal issues. If a male thinks he could have gotten someone pregnant he may register through the state paternity registry or Putative Father Registry. The majority of the states in the US provide a public registry, usually administered by the state's Department of Vital Records. A man who believes he is the father of a child can register and claim to be the father of the child and agree to be financially responsible for the care of the child. The purpose of the registries is to allow a man to register so that he will be provided notice in the event the child is placed for adoption or the state takes the child away from the mother. Let's say, for example, that a woman gets pregnant and the partner learns of it, wasn't aware of it, didn't agree with it or it just caused a wedge in their relationship and then they ultimately broke up. Now, the woman finds herself in a dire situation where she needs money and assistance. She may try to get child support from the person that impregnated her. Or, she may try to place the child for adoption without providing legal notice to the potential father. This could lead to custody issues. While people do take desperate measures you need to be aware of the consequences of those choices. Don't do something without thinking it through.

Receiving Help from a Willing Male That You Know

Another situation is when a friend helps out with getting you pregnant. Artificial insemination is a wonderful option for friends. You know their family history and it reduces some risk factors. In this case, the male enters into an agreement where his sperm is being donated, but there is no ongoing responsibility unless all parties want there to be, and they all agree to that.

Getting to Baby: Artificial Insemination Story

I have a colleague and friend who is a single woman. She is in her 40s and has not found the right man to marry. She's afraid that she may not ever find the right man to marry even though that's something she really wants in her life. She also wants children in her life.

She doesn't, at this age want to wait until she finds the right man in order to create her family. She has a good, close male friend who is also not married and does not ever plan to get married. She asked him to help her situation and he said he would. He contributed sperm. She got pregnant and now has a child. He acts more like an uncle. The child is going to grow up knowing him because he remains good friends with the mother.

This situation worked out because they communicated and defined what that relationship was going to be, what his role and involvement would be. They used the process of artificial insemination where he donated his sperm. In these situations, you can have a child fairly quickly assuming that the artificial insemination process works. In the case of the woman above, she didn't have to pay for his sperm like she would if she had bought sperm from a clinic.

Put it All in Writing: The Importance of a Contract

Using fresh sperm from someone you know who's readily available and can go make their deposit when you're ready to receive it, clinically or otherwise, can be more successful and affordable than using frozen sperm. However, legal issues could arise such as custody, child support and discrepancy over what the relationship with the child would be. Therefore, it is important to have a written agreement before beginning the process even if it's a friend.

Whenever you engage in a relationship with another person, make sure that you have paperwork including contracts and a statement of intent. Have your lawyer review these documents. A lawyer consultation for one hour is so much less expensive than lawsuits down the road.

With artificial insemination, there are the informal ways of finding the willing participant, which include intercourse and friends who donate their sperm (which you can either inseminate at home or you can use physician assisted artificial insemination.) With regard to physician-assisted artificial insemination, the couple would go to the physician, which is normally your OBGYN or fertility clinic. Remember, that it is not legal in some states for anyone other than a licensed physician to administer or perform artificial insemination. Again, do your research and consider consulting a lawyer in your area beforehand just to be safe.

Getting the Sperm You Want

There are two known ways to get sperm. You can get it from a donor such as a friend or another family member who has agreed to help or you can use an anonymous donor, which involves purchasing the sperm directly from a sperm bank.

That in itself is an interesting process. *How do you select the sperm you want?* Sperm banks have websites with profiles of the available sperm donors. What you see in that profile is their height, weight, eye and hair color, SAT scores, IQ scores and also their family history.

There are hundreds of profiles to go through. You can narrow your search. When we were looking for sperm the first time and were using fertility treatments, we sat down and asked each other, "What must this sperm donor absolutely have for you? What must they absolutely have for me?"

We decided that if we were using my egg, then wanted a sperm donor that had the characteristics of my partner so that hopefully, the child would look like one of us or a combination of us. That was important to us. We both have green eyes, so we chose a sperm donor that had blue or green eyes. We both have light brown hair so we chose a sperm donor with light brown to blond hair. My partner has curly hair so we chose someone with curly or wavy hair.

Height was very important to us because I am only 5'3". I always wanted to be taller. There are also a lot of successful traits with people who are tall. Basketball is one of my favorite sports, so I'd like to envision my children playing basketball some day. Then, there were medical issues like: *How old were their parents or grandparents when they passed away? What did they die of? Are there any genetic predispositions such as asthma, schizophrenia, alcoholism, etc.?* While it seems daunting, it became a really fun and bonding process between Jennifer and me. We would stay up for hours looking at these profiles saying, "Yes, he looks great; no, let's knock him off."

When we selected our sperm donor we had to consider issues that were important to us and should be considered by others going through the same process.

Here are some questions to consider:

1. Do you want a sperm donor that had chosen to have their identity released when the child is 18, so that child can then

look for their sperm donor and try to develop a relationship or at least meet them?

2. Or, do you want a sperm donor that says no to the identity release question?

Those are very personal choices and each person in a couple may differ on what their desires are. My partner did not want identity release, but I didn't care. It didn't matter to me one way or the other, so we chose to respect her feelings. That is just one of the questions you have to consider in addition to all of the physical characteristics.

You can buy information where the sperm donor is asked certain questions. You actually get their answers to things like: *What is your favorite food? Favorite color? Why are you donating sperm? What would you like to tell this couple if they're successful?* You get to see part of their personality through their answers.

Some sperm banks will also provide a picture when that donor was a child, like when they are three years or younger, so you can see some of the features. Some sperm banks will provide an audio of that donor answering questions so you can hear the person's voice. All of those things were important to us, so we budgeted for them so that we could compare and decide among our top three candidates.

That is how you select who will be your sperm donor. In some places, you go to the location and look in a book at profiles. With the Internet, it's readily available. That's how I would recommend doing it because you can go through multiple sperm bank websites and cut out the time you spend looking. You can sit and do it together. In our case, we had a lot of fun.

Deciding How Much Sperm to Buy

When you're buying sperm, how much would you buy? It depends.

1. How many children do you plan to have in your future?

2. Check with the physician or clinic handling your insemination and ask how many vials do they require you to buy? It also depends on how much is available on that particular sperm donor.

We have friends that were going through the process of selecting sperm. They wanted to make sure they had all the sperm from this sperm donor to try to minimize the chance of them having half-siblings out there. They bought up all his vials of sperm (of course the sperm donor could deposit more sperm which other couples could purchase, increasing the chance for half siblings again) . That was not as much of a concern to Jennifer and I, so we bought just what our clinic told us to buy, which was two vials of sperm.

The other thing to know about with regard to buying sperm is sperm quality. That is designated by the clinic that accepts the sperm and also the fertility clinic that is going to be doing the procedure. There is what's called: 'cleaned and uncleaned' sperm. Uncleaned does not mean that it's dirty, it just means that it hasn't gone through some of the filtering that's required for certain procedures.

Artificial Insemination (AI): In Vitro Insemination (IVF) and Intrauterine Insemination (IUI)

With artificial insemination it's better to use *washed sperm* (separating the sperm from the semen) because *unwashed sperm* (sperm and semen not separated) can cause severe cramping.

One frequently asked question is, *"How many times do you have to do this procedure until it's successful?"* There is no set answer. There are certainly averages, and that is why it is so important to set your limits to how many times you're going to try artificial insemination before you select another method to get pregnant. Set your limits before you begin.

The average success rate is 10-15% per cycle or pregnancy occurs generally by the third or fourth attempt, but that is an average. It is certainly not set in stone.

We have friends, a lesbian couple, who were trying to get pregnant, and they were using a clinic. They tried 12 times over the course of about a year and a half to two years because they were not doing the insemination every single month. Emotionally you have to take a break between failed attempts, as well as physically, to give your body time to rest.

Intrauterine Insemination (IUI)

Intrauterine Insemination (IUI) is a medical procedure performed by inserting a flexible catheter through the cervix and injecting washed sperm directly into the uterus. The success rate with IUI is between 6-26% per ovulation cycle. It is generally recommended that if you have completed four cycles without success, then you may want to consider IVF. The cost of IUI ranges from $200 - $6,000 depending on whether you use medication to assist with ovulation and have any other complications.

Physician Assisted vs. Doing it at Home?

The most common method of insemination is physician assisted. You have selected your sperm, it has been sent to your physician, and then you go to the office within a certain time period based on your ovulation and the date the sperm arrived and was washed. The physician or nurse will then inseminate the female.

Another method used frequently is at home with your partner doing the insemination. You have to have a mechanism in order to place the sperm in the appropriate location. This method is generally less expensive than going to the doctor. Some doctors' offices now offer instruments for couples to use at home as well. Again, remember that it is not legal in some states for anyone other than a licensed physician to administer or perform artificial insemination. Do your research and consider consulting a lawyer in your area beforehand just to be safe.

Tips for Artificial Insemination

Some tips for successful artificial insemination:

- Use fresh sperm versus frozen sperm.
- Stand on your head. I know that sounds crazy, but gravity does help.

A very good friend of mine that I've known since high school was a mentor of mine, and she was using artificial insemination for the third time. The first two times were unsuccessful. Her friends had been telling her all along to stand on her head after the insemination, and she was determined she was not going to do it. The third time was going to be her last try because she had set her limit. She figured she hadn't gotten pregnant already so what did she have to lose. After the insemination in the doctor's office, she stood on her head against the wall. The doctor walked in and asked what she was doing. She said: "I'm standing on my head. Do you have 15 minutes to wait?" The doctor didn't know quite how to respond to that and just left the room.

I don't know if that's why she was successful in her pregnancy that time or if it was just her time. Maybe she was more relaxed or maybe just being silly helped, but I do know she stood on her head, and I know that she has a child today. Step outside the box and do something a little off the wall, even if it means standing on your head at the doctor's office.

More on Costs, Insurance Coverage and Add-Ons

We can't talk about this without talking about the costs involved. There are two main ways to pay for artificial insemination. One is pay as you go. You buy your sperm or get sperm donated from someone you know. There are sperm storage fees typically.

If you were using the clinic, they would have your sperm. You would go in and pay your co-payments for each appointment or pay privately from your savings if your insurance is not covering it. You would pay each time you went in for an insemination. You would limit your cost based on the number of times you've set as far as how many inseminations you'll have or you can continue to go as long as you have the financial means to do so.

The other way to pay for artificial insemination that some clinics offer is a flat fee plan. That means you pay one fee no matter how many times it takes. Let's say, for example, it's $1,500. If you're successful on the first try it was $1,500. If it takes you 12 tries it still costs $1,500.

I can guarantee one thing. If you are successful on the first try, you're not going to think that you paid too much. You're going to be so ecstatic that you are pregnant on the first try that the cost will be insignificant. But, if it takes five, 10, or 12 times, you're going to be glad you paid that flat fee.

In many cases, fertility treatment, especially for non-traditional families, is not covered under insurance. That is why people choose to use less formal procedures than always going to the doctor. It is less expensive to go this route. (Again, check the law in your state to determine whether it is legal to "do it yourself.") When it does cover some of the cost, it generally only covers the diagnosis of the infertility issue and limited treatment. For gay couples, being gay alone is not an infertility issue. Just because you can't get pregnant because you don't have the egg or sperm is not an infertility issue for insurance companies so there is no diagnosis there. With that, you're just left with the treatment. You are normally paying out of pocket for that.

When you pay out of pocket, each procedure has its own charges. The clinics, sperm banks, and anyone you would need a service from are business people. They have learned the art of add-ons and up-sells. For example, IVF is a treatment, but now you are advised that if they assist in the hatching of the egg, then the procedure might be more successful. That is an add-on service. They're offering potentially better success if we pay more money.

Knowing this up front is very helpful so you can go in with open eyes. Find out what the process is and then determine what you will be willing to do so you're not sitting there hearing it for the first time in the doctor's office. If you hear that the procedure can potentially be more successful, you may decide to pay anything in the heat of the moment. Don't do that; know what the choices are ahead of time.

The costs for the medications are not generally included in the cost for fertility treatments. That is a separate cost that you pay as you order the medications. Fertility medications are expensive and are traditionally not covered through insurance. However, mail order pharmacies can be less expensive. Do the research.

With regard to the fertility treatment costs themselves, you will have to pay a certain large amount up front. Then, as you progress through the process, you have to pay more money at different stages. By the time the last procedure of fertility treatment takes place, the clinic has received its entire payment. This can all occur in a relatively short period of time (for example, paying between $15,000 - $30,000 within a three to six month period, plus medications).

There are companies that offer financing for these procedures and treatments. They provide you with a line of credit, which is like a credit card. It is important to note that the interest rates may be higher than other credit cards or loan opportunities. It can create a financial burden over time, which can then limit your future options of other methods because your financial situation is now different than it was when you started. Another reason to set your limits is so that you can keep your financial option open for other fertility options without having spent it all on this one type.

What I have observed, just by going through this process and sitting in the lobbies for a couple of years is that for the most part when you're at the age where you can afford fertility treatments your sperm or eggs have already retired which is why you're there getting the fertility treatments in the first place. People who are younger, who haven't established themselves in a career yet, generally can't afford fertility treatments. By the time you can afford the treatments, you need them. So stop worrying.

In Vitro Fertilization (IVF)

Ninety-five percent of all assistive reproductive technology procedures are performed through In Vitro Fertilization. This is a more invasive, more expensive procedure, with a high success rate. In our case we chose IVF from the beginning. We decided that we wanted a doctor's assistance and all the qualified help we could get. We wanted the best professionals, the best procedures, and the most reliable, predictable procedures.

With In Vitro Fertilization the infertility specialist physician specifically places an embryo transfer catheter and squirts the embryo(s) (fertilized eggs) into a specific location of the lining of the uterine cavity. The person who is getting In Vitro is not put to sleep and can watch the process on a computer screen (ultrasound monitor), so you know exactly where the physician is putting the catheter that holds the fertilized eggs.

They take the egg and the sperm and fertilize it outside the body, in a laboratory. When they are fertilized, the doctor will then select which of the fertilized eggs looks the strongest. They then suck that up into a little tube and put that tube into the woman and place it against the wall of the uterus area, the vaginal cavity. The hope is that once they've placed it there, it attaches to the wall and grows.

The only unpredictable part of IVF is whether the fertilized eggs will attach and grow. Sometimes it will absorb into the lining, and if that happens, you're not going to become pregnant. If it attaches, you will. For us, IVF was a more sure way of controlling the process because at the very least we knew we had a fertilized egg and then it was just a matter of attachment.

There is also a specialized procedure through IVF where the physicians can assist the embryo in "hatching," which may improve the embryos' ability to implant into the uterus. The idea, goal, and hope are that this will increase the chance of pregnancy.

Jennifer and I didn't just do the IVF; we did the more extensive procedure and requested assistive hatching. This procedure naturally costs more than the traditional IVF procedure. For us, fortunately cost was not an issue at the time so we could choose that method. If costs were a factor, we would have chosen a different method. That's important. We share this to let you know that there are different options of procedure and price even within one sub category of In Vitro Fertilization.

When you do In Vitro Fertilization, medication is required to help the pregnancy possibility. I called it "all the drugs" because there are so many necessary medications. Sometimes it just feels like we're just going to bend over and take a shot. There are multiple shots involved. There is a nurse who explains all the shots to you, and there is a video to watch. Then they bring out an orange and the orange is for you to practice giving the shot to so that you can go home later and give yourself the shot or have your spouse or partner give it to you. Let me just say that our skin is not like an orange!

The orange doesn't wince and tighten up when we give it the shot. It doesn't have a face with eyeballs that seem to ask, "Are you going to do it yet?" Just know that while it's good practice in the clinic, it all changes when you get home. It is something that you can do and is necessary if you're going to use this process.

With heterosexual couples, the female is taking the drugs and hormones, thus, all the shots that are taken throughout the day. With lesbian couples, if we choose to and depending on the process we decide to use, we can actually share in that pain.

When we did IVF, Jennifer and I decided that we would use my eggs, which means that we had to grow a super amount of them that the doctor could then extract. It is a surgical procedure where they make a small incision through your abdomen into the sac where the eggs are held. Then the eggs are vacuumed out. There are certain drugs that the person who's harvesting eggs needs to take to manifest a large number of eggs.

Then the person in whose body the fertilized egg is going to be transferred also has to take medication to prepare her body to accept the egg. If it is the same woman who is harvesting the eggs as well as accepting the eggs, then she has to take all of the medication. In our situation, I created and harvested the eggs and Jennifer was going to accept them.

In a way, she was my surrogate even though we're in a relationship. She needed to take certain medications to prepare her lining so it would be nice and thick and inviting for that fertilized egg to attach to it. So, we shared the pain. It was a wonderful experience because we were able to bond over the shots, the pain and also in the experience of both being physically involved in the process of creating that child.

Possible Hormonal Effects to Look Out For

With all of those medications, it's important to know that the hormones become raging and affect so many areas of our lives, both positively and negatively. For example, some of the hormones that the female takes will create a stronger desire for sexual relations. Look forward to that.

On the other hand, there can be severe mood swings like you've never seen before. If your partner or wife has ever had PMS in the way that we all think of PMS, these kinds of medications can create a behavior like PMS on steroids to the nth degree. So while this can be a stressful process that can make you tense, understand that kind of mood swing is created by the medication. It's nothing personal. Find your own space, hide for a while and let the medication do what it's supposed to do, and realize there may be a child at the end of this.

There are also other possible side effects to the medication other than your partner wanting more sex or just wanting to bite your head off. Some possible side effects, as I affectionately call it, include "the moles in our lives."

Getting to Baby: In Vitro Fertilization Story

There is one particular medication that I needed to take for the harvesting of the eggs. It said on the bottle and probably on the print out, that it could create moles on your body. I wound up having to go through the process twice. I thought everything was fine with no side effects. I didn't have any headaches and I didn't become moody or any of the other possibilities that a doctor will tell you about before you start taking these medications.

We had done the process and everything was good. I noticed that I was starting to get a few moles here and there, generally around the area where I was given the shots—in my abdomen. They were little pinpoint red spots that I knew would develop into moles at some point. And they itched.

I really like massages so I decided I wanted to get a massage at a traditional Korean bathhouse a while back. Their massages are not quite like the massage you would get at the spa in the upscale part of your town. It was what they call a body scrub. You're in this open bay with 12 different slippery plastic beds that they put you on. There are no dividers between anybody. You're totally naked. There is a female only side and a male only side, fortunately.

This Korean woman started to scrub me with this mud-like material that has very big granules in it. She scrubbed and scrubbed, and it hurt but I was mortified because I was in this room with so many other people.

She asked me at one point as she was scrubbing my back if I was okay. Well, I was in the military; I'm a tough girl and I felt like I could take it. I told her I was fine. I had no idea what was going on other than it felt like she was rubbing my skin off. I assumed that's what this was supposed to be. It was called a scrub, after all.

After she finished with the scrub, I went to shower. As I was taking my shower, I noticed that people were really looking at me and wondered why. I turned around to continue soaping myself up and as I looked at my back in the mirror, there must have been over 1,000 little pinpoint moles that I could not normally see but for the fact that this woman had scrubbed the tips off! I just didn't realize that I had all these moles created by the hormones that I was taking for the IVF procedure because I had not had these before. I did feel them, once I was made aware. They had never concerned me before because I couldn't really see them. It was extremely obvious when they were bleeding down my back because the tips had been rubbed off.

Bottom Line: Be aware that with IVF and with any other procedures where you have to take medication in order to produce fertility, there are probabilities and possibilities that there are and can be side effects. I feel very fortunate that moles were the only side effect that I received. Know what they are so you can either decide if you're willing to accept them or decide what your plan would be if you develop any of those side effects so you can deal with it and are not shocked about them later.

Multiple Medical Appointments: How to Prepare Yourself

When going through the fertility treatment process, you will have to have multiple medical appointments. Be prepared for this emotionally. You will be physically examined frequently. You will be sitting in the lobby with other people who have infertility issues. You may feel exposed or discouraged. However, you begin to see the same faces over and over and discouragement can lead to encouragement.

For me, there was a calming effect to it because when I looked around the room, I would create what other people's lives were like. It was a small escape from my own life. It was also reassuring that others are going through the same issues we were going through.

While I people watched, I tried to determine who the husband and wife were. *What was the issue? Did they have a good relationship? Were they communicating with each other like when we had to when we were planning a baby?* You'd be surprised at how many couples sit there waiting to be called for their appointment and one is on their iPhone texting the whole time and the other is reading a magazine. There is just no communication whatsoever. I felt that some level of warmth and communication, especially when you're sitting in the lobby about to have a procedure would be heartwarming.

You have to be comfortable knowing that others could be watching you too. While you may all be in the same boat, you also may not be. In some clinics, like ours, we had people like us who were trying to get pregnant, both women and men. Some of the men were there to contribute sperm. Some were not doing it for their own partners or spouses; they were doing it because they got paid to do so. You could have different people with different interests in the same lobby. Recognize that beforehand.

Success with Fertility Assistance in 12 Months or Less

Despite what we went through, we do believe it is possible to have success with fertility assistance in 12 months or less, even on a shoestring budget. We know multiple couples that have used IVF, who have had their children in 12 months or less using the procedure and didn't have to spend the larger amounts of money that many people spent, including ourselves.

A lesbian couple that we know used a known sperm donor so they did not have to pay for the sperm. The donor lives close to the couple so there weren't any travel expenses to coordinate their schedules or doctors visits. Also, another benefit of that is that they knew the medical and family history. With physician assistance with artificial insemination using fresh sperm, they were successful on the first try.

That result may not be common. The average is between the third and fourth try through artificial insemination, but they were successful on the first try and nine months later they had a healthy baby that went term. They then chose to use the same process for their second child and were successful on the third try of insemination and that child was early by two and a half months. Not that you want your child to be early just so you can do it in 12 months or less. Of course, you want a full term baby when that result can be reached, but their child was early. They used artificial insemination two times and both times were able to do it at very low cost and have children in less than 12 months from when they started.

With regard to the IVF process, if you have set your budget and your time limit on how many times you'll do that, you can also be successful in creating your child in 12 months or less.

Action Steps That Can Be Taken Now:
Finding the Right Doctor and Clinic
● ●

There are some steps you can take while pursuing your options.

1. **Do research on where the fertility clinics are in your area that specialize in artificial insemination and In Vitro Fertilization.**

2. **Talk to your OBGYN and ask if they assist with fertility treatments. Many of them will do artificial insemination.**

3. **Talk to your friends and co-workers or other family members to get recommendations on certain facilities and/or doctors for these procedures.**

In our experience, we preferred personal recommendations over individual websites.

You'll learn a lot by talking to people. Everyone knows someone who has had an infertility issue, that at some point have talked about it. When I talk about researching clinics and doctors in your area, this should take no more than two to four weeks to get a sense as to what's available in your area. Get recommendations. People are more than willing to share their opinions with complete strangers, especially online. There are forums with people who want to complain about doctors and people who want to brag on their providers, so I recommend you look for those forums.

Don't be shy; ask everyone. When we were going through this process, I would talk to my hairdresser. Everybody talks to their hairdressers, because they know everything. Your goal is to have a child so the more people that you tell, the more people can help you get closer to your goal.

4. Set a date to interview at least two different clinics.

Again, interview at least two places, which will minimize your regrets. Every clinic has issues. You just need to do your due diligence ahead of time so you can be comfortable with your choice. You wouldn't buy a car without test-driving it and choosing a doctor for one of the most important decisions you'll ever make—which is having a child— you shouldn't buy that without at least interviewing them.

5. Compare costs, apples to apples not apples to oranges.

If someone says the entire cost is a flat fee of (x) and then you have another place that says the medical procedure is this, if you have this other procedure it's that plus the medication, make sure you can equate those different types of pricing so you can truly compare them.

Ask them if there have been any price increases in the last two years, so you can get a sense of what that may be in the future. This is especially important if you are not starting at the beginning of the year. For example, if you start in July, but you are still going through the process into the next year, you need to know if your price will be locked in or if there could be a price increase.

Decide what procedure you'll use and how many times you will go through that procedure before you want to consider an alternate route. Set your budget. We recognize that we're not all wealthy. We do have limits and you will need money even after the baby is born so don't spend it all on the procedure. You'll need it for the baby and the things they need. Tell a friend or family member whom you can trust, to hold you accountable to the number of times that you set and to your budget. It's okay to put it on paper, but if you're the only one that knows it, you can scratch that out and put another figure and continue to scratch that out until you either run out of money or at some point you're successful, regardless of the cost or the procedure and what that could potentially do to your body.

More Action Steps to Consider
When Looking for the Right Fit
• •

Because they want children so bad, people will schedule a consultation with only one place. Everything sounds good and you fall in love with the possibilities that you stop doing your due diligence. So before making any decisions, go to at least two different clinics and compare their pricing and processes; see if you can meet the physicians or their nurses so you can be sure your personality mixes well with them.

1. Assess their Personality

The reason we chose the first place we used for our IVF was that we got a recommendation from a fertility lawyer who handles the contract end. We asked them to tell us the personalities of the doctors, because this lawyer knew the doctors. We chose a female doctor that was no nonsense, not someone all bubbly and flowery who would sugarcoat everything. We wanted someone who would tell us what we needed to know, someone who was more streamlined and who would do the procedure. We appreciated that. Personality is important because you have to be comfortable through the process. When someone is examining you regularly, you've got to be comfortable with them.

2. Ask what their Success Rate is

You do not need to know what the national average success rate is but what their clinic success rate is and also what that individual doctor's success rate is. At the second fertility clinic, we went to the specific doctor that had the highest success rate within that firm.

3. Check the Clinic's Legal Documents

If you're in a same sex partnership, many of these clinics don't have special legal documents that fit your situation. The documents are designed for heterosexual couples where the couple cannot have a child because either the sperm is not accessible/usable or because the egg is not usable, so they have these documents that relate to husband and wife. You cannot use forms that relate to husband/wife, so the documents have to be re-designed if the clinic doesn't already have them re-designed.

In our situation, the first clinic we went to did not have paperwork that worked for us, so we paid our lawyer to re-design it for us, which actually benefitted the clinic because then they could use them repeatedly, after we were gone. Ask about that from the beginning.

4. Ask What Type of Bank and Products Are Offered

Does the clinic you're using have a sperm bank, egg bank or an embryo bank? If you need any of those types of products, it may be best to use a clinic that also offers those.

5. Remember to Be Patient and Communicate

When I talk about our second IVF experience later on, I'll talk specifically about how we chose a fertility clinic specifically with an egg bank because we were looking for an egg donor. Those are the types of things that when you're starting to do your research that you would want to specifically pay attention to.

I would highly recommend you go back and re-read Chapter 1 and communicate with your partner about everything. All the issues that could come up, the feelings you have about those issues and if you find that either you or your partner is just agreeing with what the other person is saying, then step back and ask them how they really feel about this. It's important for both people to have a voice and to be able to express that.

This is an every day activity, which means you don't sit down for four hours and try to hash everything out because you'll get exhausted. It's something that you can incorporate into your daily communication, your daily lives and then it's something you can look forward to.

6. Stay Focused: Feng-Shui Tip

I truly believe in energy and how it affects our lives both inside our bodies and out. In our house we have what we call the abundance corner. Everything we want to bring into our lives we put all of our intentions into that corner. If you don't know about Feng Shui, we recommend you research it to determine if you would want to incorporate it into your life and getting to baby process.

I didn't spend my entire day in my abundance corner, but I focused on its importance in my goals. I focused on the other things that could help with that process, but I didn't obsess about it.

In our abundance corner, we made two bulletin boards with a ton of baby pictures, strollers, words that supported a positive healthy birth and pregnancy. We looked at it every day and confirmed our intentions while we were in that space and mood. For example, I would say in the moment: "I am blessed with a healthy child." Trust that it works and have faith that you do these things, stay at peace, and it will work.

We have friends who wanted a child so much that they couldn't talk about anything else except for everything they were doing that day to have a child. While that's important to them and we're there to support them, sometimes we want to talk about something else. Recognize in yourself if you're being that person, because that's the difference between being obsessive and being focused.

CHAPTER 4

The Adoption Option

Begin to Heal

You've made your decision
And you know it's right
But the tears keep coming
And they're hard to fight
Once you choose a couple
You will begin to heal
Sharing your hopes and dreams
And all that you feel
We have fears
And we are scared too
But we're excited
To be going through this with you

Adoption is certainly a viable choice that people consider when they can't conceive. Many people actually consider adoption as their first choice to create a family without first trying to get pregnant. Everyone knows someone who's been adopted or has had a family member or friend that was adopted. It just makes sense, when you can't have a child; you adopt a child who needs a loving home. When you cannot conceive, your mind shifts from, we want our own child, to we would love the child just as if it were our own.

One would think that there would be more than enough children to adopt with the number of teen pregnancies and with other women who have unplanned pregnancies, but there are large numbers of couples and individuals who cannot have their own children. So while we focus on the number of children that may be available, there are large numbers of couples and individuals who can't have them for various reasons.

With the laws available to us, many teens and women choose to have abortions rather than place their child for adoption. Unless you're in that situation, you don't know why someone would choose abortion over adoption. I've tried to get answers on everything in the process of getting to a baby to understand the mindset of people as to what their choices are.

Some women do not feel they can place their child in the hands of another couple and not know if that couple is truly going to take care of the child. Some women can't cope with knowing there's a child out there that they will not have a relationship with or having that child wonder why they "gave them up" for adoption. I wouldn't begin to be able to explain all the reasons why some people choose to abort, but I do know that the number of abortions in the U.S. far outweigh the number of available adoption situations in the United States.

There's also the situation where children are available for adoption, but couples do not choose them; they're considered the unwanted children. These are children that are born addicted to drugs such as crack, meth or heroine or babies that are born with disabilities and older children. You'll see children in the foster care system who are available for adoption, but because they're over a certain age or have disabilities, couples don't want to adopt them. Adoptive parents may not want to deal with the issues that can come with children who have been in foster homes because of the perception and possibility of the lack of bonding, behavior issues, and other matters of concern.

So, couples can wait years to adopt a child. It's mostly because the majority of couples want an infant without any possibility of disabilities or having had drugs in their system when they were born. There aren't as many of these babies readily available as the media portrays, compared to the number of couples seeking the adoption.

Different Types of Adoption

There are many different types of adoptions. The categories include "independent" or "agency" facilitated adoptions which then can either be open, semi-open, or closed.

Closed Adoptions

Historically, the most common type of adoptions was private adoptions. These adoptions may have historically been called: closed adoptions, confidential adoptions or secret adoptions. These adoptions are traditionally brought forward with an attorney that focuses on adoption law. A female who is pregnant may reach out to an adoption lawyer and let them know that she is pregnant and wants to place her child for adoption. The attorney would seek prospective parents to adopt the child through their own networking system or via agencies that do private/closed adoptions, or through an adoption facilitator.

With these adoptions, the parents adopting the child do not get to know who the birth mother is. They may get some medical history and limited information with regard to why the child was placed for adoption, but they will rarely see a picture of her or know her name, and she may not know the prospective parent's information either. The birth mother will get limited information about the adoptive parents but certainly not their names or where they live. Generally, there is no communication between the parties through private adoption.

There are some exceptions to the general rules. If the birth mother wants to place her child for adoption and knows someone that wants to adopt her child, they too can go through the private system. This means they are using a lawyer vs. an agency. All the processes take place privately in that, it is lawyer-assisted. Normally that's in the situation where a relative, friend or someone at church finds a couple that they know.

There are agencies that can assist with adoption and through the agencies they can do closed adoptions, as well. Religiously affiliated agencies are some of the most commonly used. How this can work is that the birth mother would hire the agency to match that child with prospective parents. If you are prospective parents and you have also hired that agency, you would be considered. In this case, it is normally those who have been waiting on the list the longest who will get that child. First come, first served.

In a closed adoption, you're not matching the couple with a baby based on any kind of traits, personality or anything that is similar between the birth mother and prospective parents. Generally with closed adoption, the prospective parents find out that they are the chosen one after the birth of the child. It's a quick process from when you find out that there's a prospective child to when you actually have the legal ability to be a parent to them. You may have been in the system waiting for a long while, but once you're notified, closed adoption can proceed very quickly.

Closed/private adoptions, in the traditional sense, are very rare today. Generally, information is shared and the birth mother, not the attorney, makes the placement decision based upon prospective parent profiles she reviews provided by the attorney or an agency.

More on Closed Adoption

A disadvantage of a closed adoption is that the prospective parents may know very little about the family history of the birth mother, the reason for the adoption in some cases, so there's no way to reach out to that person to develop any kind of relationship. A child may grow up wondering. "Why? Why was I thrown away? Why was I given up? Why couldn't my mother take care of me? Why didn't she love me enough to keep me?" This is something we hear regularly.

Unless you've been in the situation of having to place a child for adoption, you may not understand what a difficult decision it is for a woman. The choice to do that versus having that child live in a situation where she knows she cannot personally provide for the child in a positive or healthy environment is a choice of love. In a closed adoption, the child may never get to know that, other than if the prospective parents share and support that. Some adoptive parents in a closed adoption situation choose not to tell the child of the adoption. This is not recommended and can have adverse affects on the child.

There are some advantages to closed adoptions. There are no uncomfortable meetings between you and the birth mother. You don't have to worry about what you say or don't say or what you ask or don't ask. Everything is taken care of through the agency or attorney. You can express all your fears and concerns or questions to the agency as opposed to the prospective parent or birth mother.

Semi-Open Adoption

Through the semi-open process, agencies are still generally involved. It can be done with an attorney, but it's normally through an agency where the adoptive parents have hired an agency to help them do everything necessary to adopt a child, which includes getting a completed home study. They'll help you with marketing yourself, which includes a "Dear Birth Mother" letter. This is you writing a letter to a birth mother explaining who you are, where you live (not specifically, just in the region), why you desire to have children and why you're better than every other person who desires to have a child.

When the agency receives information from a birth mother that she's pregnant, they will match the birth mother's profile with what the prospective parent's profile is. The agency sends the information on the prospective parents to the birth mother, who then looks over the various profiles and chooses the one she'd like to adopt her child. All communication goes through the agency. This includes all letters between the adoptive parents and the birth mother, even after the birth, up until the child is 18 years old. All letters between the parties go through the agency, which passes them on to the recipient. For the most part, in these semi-open cases, everyone agrees that the birth mother will get pictures up until the child is 18, if that's what the birth mother wants.

Throughout this time, the birth mother and adoptive parents may never know each other's full names. They may be on a first name basis only. They may not know where the other one lives, whether it's in state, out of state, in the same city or a different city.

With the semi-open procedure, the disadvantages are that there's no real relationship being built between the adoptive parents and the birth mother. You may be introduced to the situation when the birth mother is six months pregnant, so you're waiting throughout the entire pregnancy, however long that may be, without being able to communicate with her, to get a sense for yourself if you think this is going to be a successful situation or a situation that's right for you.

You may want to know something right away, but because you have to go through the agency, which then has to get to the birth mother, there could be a delay in communication.

On the positive side of semi-open adoptions, you do get to know something about the person who's pregnant. You are able to see the medical information from the point you are selected with on-going hospitalization, doctor's visits, etc. That can make you feel more comfortable. You feel elated that this birth mother chose you, so you feel some level of bonding.

You also get the opportunity to choose the birth mother. When the birth mother chooses your profile from all she's been presented with, you can decide whether you do or don't want this baby, because you know a little more about the situation from the agency. Not everyone who goes through adoption wants an on-going relationship with the birth mother. There are a lot of people that have insecurities about the birth mother changing her mind, even though legally she cannot after finalization.

There may be that fear of, "What is the relationship going to be between her and my child? Is the child going to be confused that she's the mother or am I the mother?" It can lead to insecurities with regard to an on-going relationship. Semi-open adoption helps with that because everything goes through the agency so it can shelter that fear for a while.

Open Adoption

The other end of the spectrum is a full, open adoption. That's where a birth mother selects an individual or a couple that she wants, from looking through profiles usually, to raise her child. When she picks them, the adoptive couple gets approval through the state where they live to be able to adopt this child. A disadvantage of open adoption could be that the birth mother may truly be in your life forever, because you know her, you've had communication and have probably seen each other in person. This is reality because she is the birth mother of your child.

Another adverse situation with open adoptions is that your dear birth mother letter is presented to many potential situations. You've created this wonderful letter, and you're working with an agency that is going to present that to potential birth mothers, but while they're presenting your letter they're also presenting 10, if not hundreds of other letters to the same person. A pregnant woman or girl who's making this decision to place her child, which is not a light decision, can become overwhelmed with the number of available couples and their profiles to look through.

There is also the stress of waiting for your phone to ring if you're an adoptive couple because you've put yourself out there and from there it's a waiting game. Generally, you've gotten a separate phone number, a toll-free number, because you may be marketing to potential birth mothers across the United States. You need a way for that person to communicate with you, so you set up a separate email and phone number. You're just waiting for the phone to ring, thinking to yourself: *Why isn't my phone ringing? We're a good-looking couple, and we have so much to offer a child. Why aren't they calling me?* You race home every day to look at your phone messages or pick up your cell phone to check it every 15 minutes to make sure you didn't miss a call. That can be nerve-racking.

With the semi-open adoption process or the open adoption process, there is always a risk that the birth mother could change her mind. You've established this relationship, everything seems to be going well, you really get to know this person and she gets to know you and then, for whatever reason, she decides to parent that child. Then, you not only feel the loss of that child, the loss of the expectation of being parents, but then you start to think: *Was it something I did or said? Why didn't she like me? What did I do?* Worse yet, you start blaming your partner for what they said or didn't say, which then can create disharmony between you as a couple. (To learn about our personal experience with this, please go to Chapter 7.)

You also never truly know what a birth mother is looking for when she's looking to place her child with a couple. You have to decide what to put in the birth mother letter to make you look better than everybody else, but you just never know what she is looking for, it's all very personal. I heard a story where one couple put a picture of their home on their birth mother letter showing the kind of house they lived in. A birth mother chose them specifically because the home looked like the home the birth mother had grown up in. It was a positive experience for her growing up in a home like that. So in that case, it wouldn't have mattered what I would have put in my birth mother letter, because she based her decision on the photo of the house.

The Importance of a Birth Mother Letter

Having knowledge that little things can mean a lot, we chose to put a lot of personal information in our birth mother letter. We wanted twins, so we highlighted the fact that Jennifer is a twin. We were hoping that if there was a birth mother out there that was either a twin herself or was having twins, it would help her pick us over others because Jennifer was a twin.

We also included in our birth mother letter that I'm from Texas and Jennifer is from Kansas and we now live in Georgia, so if there was any kind of connection to any of those states that might form a bond between us and her. You really just don't know, but going in with a positive mindset can help you trust the process and let it unfold naturally.

Requirements for Most Adoption Options

A home study, background check and medical clearance are generally required for all adoptions, including second parent adoptions. State laws vary widely and there are many exceptions. It is advisable to contact an attorney specializing in adoption law in your state to determine what is required. If you are using an adoption agency, they can advise you on the requirements.

Through all of the adoption options, whether closed, semi-open and open adoption, the adoptive couple has to go through the home study, background check and medical clearance. The adoptive couple compiles their marketing package, which includes a Dear Birth Mother letter, which usually includes pictures of themselves with children. If they don't have their own children, they can be pictured with other children. And finally, you'll include stories about who you are. It's all about positioning yourself so that you look like the best potential couple to raise that person's child.

Set a Strong Foundation and Network!

With adoption, it's about marketing and networking with those you know. When you decide you want to adopt, that would be the time to reach out to that you know. You want to start with a strong foundation first though.

Hire a Marketing or Graphic Designer

We hired a company to help us design a website, along with the birth mother letter. We highly recommend this to people going through the open adoption process. With our agency, when we first started, the letter could not be more than a front and back piece of standard 8.5x11 paper. You have to put pictures and good text, but there's not a lot of room. The agency did not regulate the website so we could put as many pages and text as we wanted. Our website was posted on-line way before our agency approved our letter. A strong birth mother letter and website could be the difference between you getting a baby or not.

Consider Google AdWords

Before our birth mother letter was approved to be included in the profiles book, we placed an advertisement on Google. If you're not familiar with how to do that, Google has AdWords that you can purchase. If you go to Google, AdWords are the sponsored links you see down the right hand side and at the top of the page when you do a search on a word within Google. So, if someone was going to search on the keyword "adoption," ads will pop up on the right hand side of a web page, and that person can click through and see what the offer is. We created a profile, and purchased some ad space on Google even before we were technically "in the book" with our adoption agency because we wanted to be very aggressive in our marketing efforts. We didn't want to rely solely on our agency to do the marketing for us.

We received a ton of calls through our Google ads. Some appeared to be scams but others were legitimate. It's exciting to get the call because it's an opportunity for you to create your family but also you get enthused that that they chose you. You need to have a list next to the phone of the topics you want to discuss and questions that you can ask so there is no dead space, otherwise you will get nervous. It's so important to be prepared with that list. Recently, couples have begun to upload YouTube videos about their desires to adopt a child, as well as blogging about it. **Important cautionary note:** It is not legal to advertise in Google or otherwise in some states. Do your research and consider consulting a lawyer in your area beforehand just to be safe. It would be devastating to adopt a child through a contact wherein your efforts were considered as "advertising" and then have that adoption become void or invalid later.

Getting to Baby: Networking Story

Our office building was being renovated for quite some time. The project's manager was a woman in her 40s. Since I was a carpenter in the Air Force we formed a bond. We talked and I realized through our communication that she had a daughter in her late teens to early twenties, which in my mind, is the perfect age to market to if I'm looking to adopt a child.

I brought my birth mother letter to her and I asked her to share it with her daughter. I explained that she might have friends in an unwanted pregnancy situation. Interestingly enough, about eight months after I shared our letter with her, I was down at the café in our building and she wanted to talk with me about the letter I gave her.

I told her she could come by my office anytime. Three days later, I saw her again and asked if she wanted to talk. She looked like she hadn't slept in days. She explained that her daughter had been pregnant, but she lost the baby, so there was no need to talk to me anymore. She told me they were going to ask me if we still wanted to adopt. This goes to show that you just never know where your connection may come from.

Use Social Media and Viral Marketing

We started Facebook and MySpace pages because of the networking opportunities. When we were going through that process, Jennifer and I were 38 years old, so we figured that a lot of people we went to high school with had children that were 16-20 years old. That is the age range where if someone has an unplanned pregnancy, they may be looking at the adoption option for placement of their child. So the sole reason we created the social media pages was to let everyone know that we were looking to adopt a child. We asked everyone that if they knew of a situation that presented itself to please let us know. Reconnecting with people whom you never thought that you would receive support from can be helpful.

Our Facebook page helped connect us with all of our high school friends and even those people we weren't friends with back then. It's an amazing thing—everyone is a friend on Facebook! We accepted every friend request that we received on Facebook.

What resulted from that was important. One of my good friends from junior high school contacted me. We had stopped being close through high school. I thought she had transferred schools. She did not transfer but was kept behind so we weren't in the same class anymore. I didn't even realize that she was at the same school as me. My school had over 4,000 people in it, so it was easy to lose touch.

We reconnected on Facebook, and she was a birth mother. Right after high school she got pregnant and knew that she was not going to be able to raise that child the way she felt it should be raised so she placed her child for adoption.

We shared with the entire Facebook world that we were looking to create our family through adoption. She emailed me and shared her story. It opened up a great dialogue and when things didn't go well for our adoption, she was there for me and supported me emotionally. We started talking on the phone, as well.

When you get calls from potential birth mothers and going through the entire adoption process, you want to know everything you can about what's in the mind of a birth mother. Realistically, everybody is different, but if you can talk to one of them, you think you have the advantage. In talking to my friend from junior high, I got information that I could not have gotten from anywhere else.

I also serve on several non-profit boards, so I gave my birth mother letters out to everybody there as well. One of the women on one of those non-profit boards had a husband who owned rental property. She talked to him about the letter. In one of his rental houses, he had a tenant that was seven months pregnant. She was not paying her rent, so he'd go out to visit her quite a bit. She had expressed to him that she needed to place her child up for adoption. Because I had given his wife one of these letters, he thought of me. The wife called me and told me about the situation, so you never know!

We also had our professionally designed website which we sent out to our entire email list—even professionally. I'm a lawyer and own my own firm. The perception is that you have to be careful on what you share, not to cross the professional/personal lines, but I have gotten to the point in my profession that I disagree with that. I do much more business and am much more successful when I do show my personal side. My clients and professional contacts were out there rooting for me once I emailed about it, keeping their eyes and ears open. This is called viral marketing and if you are looking to adopt, we highly recommend that you use it!

Which Adoption Option is Best?

In our opinion, the open adoption process is certainly the best process of the three. An advantage of open adoption is that when a birth mother chooses you as the couple, you have the absolute right to say yes or no to this situation. So, if the birth mother says: "I would like you to raise my child and become their legal parent," you can ask for more information about the medical situation, family history. You can ask if she was drinking during her first trimester, etc. If it's a situation you don't feel comfortable with or in your gut it just doesn't feel right, you can decide to pass on the situation and wait for another one.

You can base your decision on characteristics of the birth mother and possibly the birth father. You can't overlook the fact that a birth father may still be involved with the birth mother. He may still be part of the decision process as to choosing who raises their child. Also, the birth father may want an on-going relationship with that child like a birth mother through open adoption.

There are also some geographic advantages. You may look at it as a good thing that the birth mother and adoptive family live in the same state, so you can actually see each other more often. On the flip side, maybe that's not something you are comfortable with. Even with an open adoption process, the birth mother could live in Washington State and you in New York State. This way, phone calls, letters and pictures are easily exchanged and are part of your open adoption, but you also know that birth mother isn't going to come knocking on your door every other day, because geographically she would be prevented from doing so.

Another advantage is that the pregnancy may be at an early or late stage. With an early stage pregnancy, you get to be more involved from the beginning; you get to design what your relationship with that birth mother is going to be. You can agree on whether you may go to doctor's visits with her, whether she will give you sonogram pictures, how much involvement you can have along the way to support her in her pregnancy, develop the relationship between the two of you, and to start bonding with the child even before he or she is born.

If you aren't notified until the latter stages of the pregnancy, you'll still get to know a lot about the birth mother. While you get to meet each other through open adoption, you may not want a long courtship. You may not want to do everything to walk that tightrope of making sure everything is okay and that she doesn't change her mind. Sometimes a late meeting during the pregnancy is an advantage.

Depending on your exact situation, almost everything mentioned here could go either way as far as advantages and disadvantages for you, but it's important to go in knowing as much information as you can. What is an advantage for me may be a disadvantage for you and vice versa.

Adopting Internationally

We've talked about the three different types of adoption that are the most common in domestic situations, which means you're adopting within the United States and you are also a resident of the United States. However, many people choose to do international adoptions. There are some exceptions to that rule where you do get to know the birth parents, but generally, they are closed adoptions.

In 2009, the United States ratified the Hague Convention on Adoption which has significantly changed international adoption and, in general, the number of children being adopted into the U.S. from abroad. Seek knowledgeable legal counsel who can assist you with some of the issues raised below.

It's important to research what countries are legally allowing you to adopt. The most common places that used to be open to it were Russia, China and some Central and South American countries. But of late, there have been a lot of scams and fraud with regard to adoption agencies that would take prospective parent's money, tens of thousands of dollars and then have no child ready for them to adopt.

Some countries may restrict adoptions based on the age of the prospective parents, especially for males. You have to be under a certain age if you're going to adopt from certain countries. Also many countries will only allow heterosexual couples to adopt, so if you were a same sex couple, then you would have to present yourself as a single individual. Many countries will not allow single men to adopt children. That may be an issue for male couples.

You would want to run a background check on the agency you're thinking of using to determine whether or not they have committed fraud or if there are any complaints against them. With regard to international adoptions, the time it takes to do the adoption can be very lengthy. While it may seem shorter because you match with a child sooner, in many cases, it can actually take a long time to complete the process which means the child you adopt is older than you might adopt domestically.

Normally if you adopt a child from Russia, the child has already been born by the time you are matched with them. Because of the process, that child may be eight months to a year and a half before you get to bring it back to the United States. So for people who only want to adopt an infant, you will want to stick to domestic adoption in the United States. If that is not an issue for you, then international adoption may be a wonderful option. Many of the children who are in another country awaiting adoption live in what is considered an orphanage, so there may be physical or emotional issues with a child that you would want to ask about and become aware of before the child is placed with you.

When you're adopting an international child, there are certainly cultural differences that must be kept in mind. There are types of communication and self-awareness that you would want to explore. For example, will the child learn about their culture as well as yours or do you just teach them the American way? You should explore how you feel about those issues. It is also important to research how you can bond with a child who is a toddler when you didn't have an opportunity to bond with them as an infant.

Adoption Agencies and Facilitators

There are adoption agencies that are traditionally non-profit organizations. Then there are adoption facilitators who are generally, individuals, but they can be companies. They are extremely different. Adoption agencies are licensed and regulated by state law; for the most part, facilitators are not, which can leave prospective parents unprotected.

Not all agencies are created equal. Some adoption agencies are focused on the adoptive parents, the couple who wants to have a child. They'll spend a lot of money marketing to that population and their efforts are strictly focused on adoptive couples that want to have children. They charge the couple a fee to represent them and then help them complete their home study, get their background checks and do everything so they're ready to adopt a child when an available situation presents itself.

These types of agencies may have hundreds of couples as clients who are waiting to adopt a child. These agencies may be either local –

like a mom and pop agency – or they may be national where they have several different offices throughout the United States.

Important Questions to Ask When Choosing an Agency

The agency we used was national, and its headquarters was in California. What we learned, while going through the process, was that there were over 200 couples waiting to adopt a child.

Because the corporate headquarters was in California, this company spent the majority of its marketing budget to the birth mothers in that state, which could detrimentally affect the clients from other offices not located in California.

Things to consider include:

1. How large and what is the location of the agency? Where's the corporate office?
2. How do they market to birth mothers?
3. What percentage of the budget dollars is used for each location?
4. What is the agency's reputation and success rate?

Get references for the agency you're looking to use. There are so many out there. Some are excellent, some are middle of the road and some are not good at all. It's just like any other business.

There are also agencies that are focused more on the birth mother than the adoptive parents. The agency does not take any clients that are looking to adopt a child, but instead spend all their marketing money to attract pregnant women who want to place their child for adoption. They pay for a lot of the pregnancy costs of the birth mothers, which may include medical, housing, day-to-day things for which the courts allow. These types of adoption agencies frequently will use adoption facilitators to match the birth mother with a couple who wants a child.

Since these agencies don't market to the couples, they have to find couples through adoption facilitators. These agencies that focus on birth mothers have higher fees, usually between $30,000 and $50,000. If you're an adoptive couple presented with a situation with a birth mother at an adoption agency that focuses on birth mothers, you pay the full fee up front. It is non-refundable, with the possible exception of the birth mother is under the age of 18. It depends upon the policy of each agency.

Getting to Baby: Adoption Story

When we were going through adoption, we were presented with a situation from an agency that focused solely on birth mothers. The fee was $42,000. The birth mother was 17 years old, just three months shy of 18, so we did not pay the fee up front. Had we paid the fee up front and if the adoption was unsuccessful, the adoption agency would not have refunded our fee. You will, however, become a priority client so if another situation presents itself and you match that profile, you will be offered the opportunity first. There are no guarantees that you will be successful or offered a certain opportunity. Therefore, it's important to know that in advance since there's a lot of money on the line.

What is an Adoption Facilitator?

Adoption facilitators are individuals or companies that have relationships with adoption agencies focused on birth mothers. Facilitators also have relationships with prospective parents that want to adopt children. Adoption facilitators also have relationships with doctors, hospitals and lawyers who do private adoptions. When an available situation arises (meaning a birth mother is either pregnant or has just had a child), the adoption agency or a lawyer or doctor contact the adoption facilitator. Then, the adoption facilitator offers that situation to the adoptive couple by giving some basic information. The adoptive couple decides if they would like to have their profile presented to that birth mother. Then, the birth mother will review the profile. Adoption facilitators usually have anywhere from 5 to 25 clients, which is much less than the traditional adoption agency would have.

Adoption facilitators only present one to three profiles at a time to the birth mother so she isn't overwhelmed. They do not have the legal authority to actually create an adoption situation; they're just introducing two people who can take it from there through either an agency or a lawyer. Using an adoption facilitator may greatly reduce the amount of time you're waiting to adopt a child because they've developed relationships with agencies focused on birth mothers and physicians. The good adoption facilitators will limit the number of clients they accept. That way the clients are not waiting a long time for an available situation that matches their profile.

Adoption facilitators; however, are not licensed agencies. Adoption agencies must be licensed through the state where they are practicing, and they must follow certain guidelines in order to create the adoption situation. Facilitators have little to no regulation because there are no federal laws that discuss what a facilitator can and cannot do and every state has its own laws with regard to adoption. This is not intended to be legal advice. Just know that laws vary state by state and generally, there is very little oversight for adoption facilitators.

Important Questions to ask
When Choosing an Adoption Facilitator

You must do your due diligence because some adoption facilitators are scams. They will charge you a fee up front and never find an adoption situation for you because they don't have the relationships with the appropriate agencies. It's very important to ask:

1. What is their reputation and how long have they been in business? Ask for references.

2. Which agencies refer to them?

3. How many adoptions they have been involved with over the course of the past year?

Getting to Baby: Adoption Facilitator Story

When we were going through the adoption process, with our need for speed and immediate results, we hired an adoption facilitator. I learned of the adoption facilitator through a colleague of mine who was a single woman who wanted a child and she was friends with an adoption facilitator. Prior to becoming an adoption facilitator, she had spent many years conducting adoption home studies for an adoption agency.

First, I knew that she knew what the process was because she had worked for an adoption agency for many years before opening her own business. Second, she had helped with the adoption situation of my colleague and that was successful. That was my main reference and when I looked at her website, I was impressed. She had listed how many adoptions she had helped to facilitate over the last year, and it was many more than my own adoption agency had facilitated for that same period of time, so we paid for the adoption facilitator.

We wound up working with more than one facilitator. The adoption agency that had the birth mother with the child that we were adopting had a relationship with an adoption facilitator. That particular adoption facilitator did not have any couples on her list that met the profile, because this particular birth mother wanted a lesbian couple. So, the adoption facilitator that had the relationship with the adoption agency didn't have any couples to present to her. She then reached out to her friends, her network of professionals which led to our adoption facilitator that we had hired. We paid for both adoption facilitators because they both had a role in the situation. We did get a reduced fee for the original adoption facilitator that had the relationship with the agency. There could be multiple layers with hiring an agency, a facilitator, etc. You may use more than one option but knowing them is the most important thing.

Jennifer and I wish we had known about the adoption facilitators before we hired our agency. That doesn't mean we wouldn't have hired the agency because they did help us with the home study, the background check and medical check. They gave us the checklist and made sure we were doing everything appropriately. While some facilitators can assist with those checklists, we felt very comfortable having an agency. Also, whenever we had a situation present itself, if we had fears, questions or any concerns, we could simply call our agency and ask those questions. We felt like we were optimizing our opportunities by having both an agency and a facilitator. However, if you're trying to minimize costs, then you may want to choose one option over the other and if you want to shorten the length of time to become a parent through adoption, you may want to do some research on adoption facilitators.

Adoption Expenses

The large expenses associated with adoption are the agency fees. If it's an adoptive parent focused agency that's a non-profit, fees can range from $5,000 to as much as $20,000 in some states. If it is birth parent focused, and you find a child through either your agency or another adoption facilitator, you still have to pay the agency fees (that the birth mother chose to use) and those fees range from $25,000 to $50,000. The adoption facilitator fees can range from $3,000 to $12,000. My opinion is that there are some really good adoption facilitators on the lower end of that range. Just because they charge more does not mean they're better.

There are expenses to the birth mother that an adoptive parent may agree to pay for. State law governs what expenses may be paid; consult with a reputable adoption attorney to determine what is allowed. Types of expenses that come up are housing; transportation, such as a bus card or a taxi; daycare or babysitting for their children, because they may have other children they're caring for; medical expenses; and food. Other types of expenses may be permissible depending on the particular state you are in. Certainly, there can be more or fewer, but those are the most common.

Fees for an adoption facilitator vary across the United States. Ours was $3,000. Normally that is paid up front to be a priority client. Because we knew the particular adoption facilitator and she kept a very small list, and we were the only lesbian couple on it, she told us we didn't have to pay up front. She looked for a situation for us and once we matched with a child that she found for us through an adoption agency, we paid her fee.

Many of the expenses that are paid to a birth mother are paid to the agency, which then pays for the items the birth mother needs. Or the expenses could be paid directly to the birth mother, but they would need court approval. There are attorney's fees and court costs. If the birth mother does not live in the same city or state you live in, there may be travel expenses that you're paying in order to meet with the birth mother. Or, when the child is born, you may have to travel to be where the child is born and then you may have to stay there for a couple weeks until the adoption process is completed.

When it comes to paying for adoption expenses, it's generally, through your own savings. Some people borrow from family members or friends or ask for gifts. Some people who don't have those other resources available to them will get a line of credit from their house or use credit cards. Some even work second jobs. Just as we mentioned in the first part of this book, if you need additional money, the best time to work an unlimited number of hours is before you have the children. And also, remember to set and stick to a budget.

Financial Relief: Our Own Experience

We are not financial advisors and cannot give you tax advice, but through our own experience, we learned that first, there is a Federal Adoption Tax Credit when you adopt a child, even if the adoption fails. The amount of tax credit may vary depending upon the year. For example, in 2009, it was $11,560. A tax credit means that you can deduct dollar for dollar what you have spent towards that adoption. We had a few failed adoptions, two that were extremely close to completion, and we spent $13,000 with our adoption agency. We also had $3,000 with our first adoption facilitator, $1,700 on our second adoption facilitator and travel expenses to two different states where these two children were to be born.

We didn't know that we could claim those expenses towards the adoption credit, because they were failed adoptions. We went back two years to when the adoptions failed in 2008/2009 and we've claimed those failed adoption expenses. And, because we are a same sex couple and marriage is not recognized under the federal tax laws, we each were able to take advantage of the tax credit as long as we did not claim the same expenses/credit for the same child. No double dipping is allowed.

Also because we had multiple children that were presented in different situations, we were each able to choose which one we would claim the adoption credit against. That can be an advantage to same sex couples with regard to taxes. Check into claiming all the expenses for all the years that involve any successful or unsuccessful adoptions.

Consider that there are some medical expenses that you can deduct from your taxes if you itemize. If your medical expenses reach a certain amount in relation to your income, you may be able to deduct some of your medical expenses. This relates to procedures like IVF and artificial insemination, but also to the adoption process.

The Federal Adoption Tax Credit is not a permanent part of the Tax Code and is set to expire in 2012. This provision may or may not be extended beyond 2010. It is critical that you consult with a tax attorney or certified public accountant when considering making any claims under the Federal Adoption Tax Credit.

Adoption Scams and Warning Signs

Unfortunately, whether you are looking to adopt a child from the United States or another country, you must be aware that there are people scamming prospective adoptive parents. Agencies can scam by taking money from prospective parents and then never having an available situation to present. Most prevalent; however, are individuals trying to scam other individuals. The scams are generally one of two types: financial or emotional. There are red flags to assist in identifying each type.

With regard to financial scams, some red flags include: a birth mother who asks for money directly from the prospective adoptive parents the first or second time they make contact; unwilling to use or talk with an agency or the agency the prospective parents are using; avoidance of meeting the prospective parents in person; telling the prospective parents that they don't want to use lawyers or get court permission for financial expenditures.

With regard to emotional scams, birth mothers (or those posing as birth mothers) do not generally seek any financial assistance. Instead, they keep prospective parents on the phone for lengthy conversations, sharing all their troubles in an effort for the couple to feel sorry for them. The scammer will call around holidays and beg for the prospective parents to adopt the child, sometimes saying that other prospective parents changed their minds at the last minute. The scammer may indicate she has twins or the birth father has died and without him she cannot raise the child.

Fortunately there are some really good scam boards available on the internet. If you feel you have been presented with a potential scam situation, refer to the boards, explain your situation and ask if anyone has heard of this person or situation. We used the scam boards with our situation with Sharon. While we cannot confirm she was a scam, we did confirm from the scam boards that she had presented herself as available and seeking to match with couples after she had already matched with one or more.

Fun Facts about Adoption

While this book is about a serious matter, it's also important to have some fun facts in here. Many people are drawn to celebrities. Here are some that have adopted children:

Walt Disney

Babe Ruth

John Denver

Burt Reynolds

Diane Keaton

Kirstie Alley

Sharon Stone

Rosie O'Donnell

Tom Cruise and Nicole Kidman

Angelina Jolie and Brad Pitt

Sandra Bullock

Jamie Lee Curtis

People in all walks of life and in different situations have chosen to adopt children and provide a good life for them. On the other side of the spectrum is someone like Joan Crawford, who chose to adopt children and didn't provide a good life for them. It's also interesting to know how many celebrities themselves are adopted. Here's a brief list:

Marilyn Monroe

Dave Thomas, founder of Wendy's Hamburgers

President Bill Clinton

Rev. Jessie Jackson

John Lennon

Eric Clapton

Steve Jobs, co-founder of Apple

Debra Harry, lead singer of Blondie

Faith Hill

Greg Louganis, Olympic Diver

The perception can be that adopted children can grow up insecure and withdrawn because they don't know where their heritage came from. They may feel that their birth parents didn't want them, but the previous list provides a good example of adopted people that have became very successful.

The third category is birth mothers and birth parents that have chosen to place their children for adoption:

Joni Mitchell

Andy Kaufman

Kate McGrew

These are all people that we know who have been touched by adoption in one way or another. We would encourage you to watch the movie *Juno* if you are considering adopting a child. It's a movie that gives you an idea and possibly some empathy as to what the birth mother and/or birth father goes through when they have an unexpected pregnancy. It's a sweet story about a girl in high school who has intercourse with her best friend. It's the first time for both of them, and it's about what they go through when she get's pregnant. It gives a realistic view of what adoptive parents can experience, as well.

Adoption Action Steps

It is important to have action steps and one is to list the people you know who have been adopted or who have placed a child for adoption. If you think they're willing to talk about the situation, reach out and ask them if you can talk with them about their experience.

Can you walk into a pet store without crying when you leave all the puppies or kittens if you can't take one home? I'm a big animal lover, and it's very difficult for me to do that. Not that I would equate children to pets, although, many people do. I have a pet that I consider my four-legged child, but I think it tells you something about yourself. If you have strong emotions for a pet, then you may be strongly affected through the adoption process when the adoption doesn't turn out the way you would like it to.

Ask those around you who have been adopted or who have placed for adoption what they're experiences have been. Have you read any stories about adoption? There are some great books that talk about open and closed adoption, what the advantages and disadvantages are. There are books written by people who are adopted and their adoption experience. The more you can familiarize yourself with the key players and the process, the easier it is emotionally to go through that process.

Adoption Checklist

Have you:

1. Contemplated all the positive and negative consequences of adopting both domestically and internationally and made a decision that feels right for both of you?

2. Researched the agencies and asked for references?

3. Set your budget?

4. Set your timeframe of how long before doing something else, choosing another option or stopping all together?

5. Put your support system in place?

6. Are you totally committed to this method?

The reason that #6 is so important is that many people will continue to try to get pregnant while they're in the adoption process. They may match with a birth mother, they're intending to adopt this child and then they get pregnant.

Getting to Baby: Adoption Story

There was a situation that I heard of, a lesbian couple that was in the adoption process and they matched with a birth mother. After they had gone through the fertility process and became pregnant they found out that they had matched with a birth mother. They decided to continue the adoption and have the child. Now they have two children that are very close in age, not quite twins but very close in age.

That can be a strain on a relationship, on the financial budget and the whole process of the adoption, especially if the birth mother finds out that you're pregnant. She may be worried that you'll change your mind at the last minute before she can find another couple.

I view pursuing two different methods or more at the same time like the tail wagging the dog. It can be exhausting and nonproductive, yet you want to be flexible because you want that child.

I've mentioned previously that if you want a Caucasian baby with blond hair and blue eyes from a healthy 20-year old woman, expect to wait a long time. They're not as frequent as you would think and many people want that child. Be diverse in your considerations. Consider a child that may be biracial or African American. Consider adopting from a woman that may have had some alcohol during her first trimester or continued to use drugs during pregnancy. Educate yourself by speaking with physicians about the effects of alcohol and drug exposure.

Getting to Baby: Adoption Story

Friends of ours adopted a child from a birth mother who was a drug addict. The birth mother was literally going from the hospital out into the parking lot and smoking marijuana the week before the baby was born. Marijuana was the softer of the drugs that she was choosing to take while pregnant. Amazingly the baby was born with no drugs in its system whatsoever. Talk to a physician as to what the probabilities are.

Remember, don't judge the birth mother unless you too want to be judged. They have been judged generally their entire lives about something. We all have been. Feel blessed that while her situation may be unfortunate for her, it can be a good situation for you. Approach it with kind, open and loving arms and not one with judgment. Many people who choose to adopt a child come with that attitude of being judgmental.

Whether you choose open or closed adoption, choose to hire an adoption facilitator or go about the process in a more unconventional way, the more open-minded you are, the better your chances of getting to baby.

CHAPTER 5

Success with Surrogacy

"None of us knows what the next change is going to be, what unexpected opportunity is just around the corner, waiting a few months or a few years to change all the tenor of our lives." —Kathleen Norris

In a sense, surrogacy is truly just a fertility treatment with a new name. Through surrogacy, you still use artificial insemination or In Vitro Fertilization, the IVF procedures. It's the same game. There is a couple that wants to have a child but a different woman is used to do it. You're using a third person, a woman, who can carry that child for you.

Surrogacy is not an option that people jump to when they can't conceive or get pregnant to have their own children, but it can potentially save thousands of dollars and cut years off of the process of creating a family. I asked myself, "Why didn't I know about surrogacy from the beginning? After the fertility, would we have chosen surrogacy instead of adoption if we had known about it?" It's like a secret underworld.

There was a time when people used to whisper, "Hey, he's gay." Well, it's almost like that with surrogacy. Surrogacy agencies are not marketing to pull you in; there are no billboards like there are for adoption that say, "Choose surrogacy to have your children."

The people who use surrogacy, by and large, are not shouting from the mountaintops that they used another woman to help them create their family. Most people assume that you adopted a child, even through the surrogacy process.

Getting to Baby: Surrogacy Story

Even with me, I had a colleague that told me about his process and I wasn't ready to hear it—the light bulb didn't go off until our second failed adoption. I think our minds were so set on, "If we can't get pregnant we must adopt." Surrogacy didn't even enter into the equation at first.

The entire time when we *were* using a surrogate, so many people asked us when we would be adopting the child. It's not the same process, but many equate it to that.

I know that if we had been in tune to it, we could have personally saved two years of our lives and had babies sooner assuming all went the way it did with our surrogacy. We could have saved at least $25,000 to $50,000. At this point, we say, "We could have, we would have, we should have, but we didn't."

One of the reasons that I am sharing this information is that I want people to know that surrogacy is a real viable option to create a family. It's one both Jennifer and I believe in strongly, because it was our successful option. We feel we can help people go through that process and save a lot of time and money.

When you want to have a child, it's about having that child as soon as possible and not spending all of your life savings to create that family. All the other issues with regard to creating your family as far as the cost, the success rate, and emotional issues that we have already talked about are the same as going through the fertility process.

Surrogacy Agencies
• • • • • • • • • • • • • • • • • • •

There are surrogacy agencies that you can find online that have women who are already qualified to be surrogates and who are available for surrogacy. These agencies are extremely expensive. A couple should expect to pay no less than $100,000 when using an agency. While some of that fee goes to the surrogate, the majority goes to the agency.

The agency has the ready list of surrogates available. If you don't want to find one on your own, this is a way to be able to pay, have a surrogate immediately who you choose from available profiles.

Surrogates can be from all over the United States and the world. Unlike adoption, there are very limited laws on surrogacy. When you use a surrogate through an agency, there's usually no relationship between the couple and the surrogate. That can be an advantage or disadvantage depending on what level of relationship you want to have.

If there is no relationship or if that surrogate lives across the world, that can limit your ability to partake in the process, go to doctor appointments and things like that. All surrogates who go through credible and ethical agencies have to meet certain requirements.

The surrogate must be under a certain age, has to have their own children already, their body fat index must be less than a certain number, and they have to disclose any mental health issues or any medications they're taking or have taken. It is a screening process that the agency does for two reasons. First, it ensures the likelihood of success with regard to carrying a child to term and second, it confirms the surrogate's choice not to parent that child.

"Want Ad" Websites
• • • • • • • • • • • • • • • • • • •

If you don't go through an agency and want to do this informally on your own, which is the way we did it, there are surrogacy "want ad" websites. These are websites on which surrogates have the opportunity to put an advertisement on and intended parents can put an advertisement on it with the hope that they'll match with each other.

We went to a website called www.surromomsonline.com. We looked through the available postings by potential surrogates. There were also a lot of postings by potential prospective parents. Looking at those is important because you want to see what people are saying and how they are advertising themselves.

Most of the ads by surrogates who are looking for couples focus on helping Christian families or gay men, but not lesbians. "Christian families" is code for saying "married, heterosexual couples."

There are a lot of surrogates who want to help gay men. There wasn't anyone who advertised that they would help lesbians. When I contacted several of the people who seemed to be more liberal in their altruistic ways, I mentioned we were a lesbian couple and many of them said, "Huh? I hadn't thought of that."

When I inquired further, they said they wanted to help a couple that could just never have children on their own. The perception is that lesbians can have their own children. There is generally no prohibition about advertising like there is with adoption. This is one indication that this process is very different from adoption.

At these "want ad" websites, there is generally a forum for discussion. There may be an intended parent discussion board so they can talk to each other and ask questions such as, "Have you heard of this other surrogate?" "Are you having issues with your surrogate?" "How is this working out?" etc.

Then there are the surrogacy discussion boards as well. When surrogates are going through the process, they tend to group and follow each other. It's a support system for surrogates, which is very important to have.

This is an informal process, which means you've got to create your own contracts to formalize the relationship. You must do everything to make sure this is going to be successful on your own because you don't have an agency that is working for you.

Know the Different Types of Surrogacy

Whether you're using an agency for surrogacy or doing it informally, there are two different types of surrogates.

1. Traditional carriers

2. Gestational carriers

There is a huge difference between the two. You may ask yourself, why would you care? You just want a baby. You care because the laws and the emotional aspect are very different between the two.

A traditional carrier is a woman who uses her own egg that is fertilized generally by a husband's sperm or the intended parent's sperm. For a gay male couple, it would be one of their sperm selections. For a heterosexual couple, it's the sperm of the husband. For a lesbian couple, we would be buying the sperm and inseminating the traditional carrier so that she gets pregnant using her own egg.

In that situation, you identify what sperm you're going to use; you wait for the surrogate to have her menstrual cycle because everything is based on her body cycle. Then you would most likely use artificial insemination because it is the less expensive option, but In Vitro Fertilization can be used where the surrogate harvests her eggs and then they are extracted and fertilized outside the body and then put back in. Artificial insemination is the most common method for traditional surrogacy.

Because the surrogate is using her own egg, she has a biological connection to that child, so there is a higher risk that she may change her mind and want to parent that child. And, she has a legal right to do so because it's her egg and she's the mother. By law, that child is hers. The only thing you have is a contract between the two of you that she will place that child with you as the parent.

If she breaches that contract, it's a contract claim, legally speaking, and the only thing the intended parent can recover under a breach of contract claim is actual damages which means the money spent out of pocket that was incurred because of the contract such as any medical or housing expenses you paid. You would not be able to recover any emotional damage, such as pain and suffering or the time lost of not being pregnant because the woman changed her mind and decided to keep this child.

That's very different from a gestational carrier, which is a surrogate who uses the egg of another person. Generally, it's the wife of the couple. This process is through IVF, In Vitro Fertilization, where the wife of the couple harvests her own eggs, and then it is fertilized in the Petri dish with either the husband's sperm or with other sperm. Then the fertilized egg is put into the surrogate.

Getting to Baby: Surrogacy Story

In our case, we used a gestational carrier and purchased donor eggs. We had already found out through our fertility treatment process that I don't have very many eggs and they are weak. When we talk about sperm, we talk about clean and dirty sperm. When we talk about eggs, it's strong or weak eggs.

We also found out that Jennifer may not produce eggs at all so we didn't want to go through a bunch of testing to determine that for sure. We were very happy with the fact that we could purchase eggs. We used anonymous eggs, fertilized them with sperm and used the IVF process to transfer them into our surrogate so she's a gestational carrier, not using her own eggs.

That process works well because after you fertilize the eggs they're transferred into the gestational carrier three to five days after fertilization. Shortly thereafter, you know if you're pregnant. There is no legal issue as to who the parent is at that point because it's not the gestational carrier's egg.

Seeking a Surrogate on Your Own

It's a personal choice as to who you're looking for and what to look for in a surrogate, but there are certain things that are important to remember. You want to use similar guidelines to what the agencies use.

1. It's important that she already has her own children.

The likelihood of her changing her mind is less when she feels that her family is complete. You also want someone who you can talk with naturally and who you enjoy being around. In the beginning of this process, you are meeting with a woman who is not yet pregnant. The full term pregnancy is nine months away so this is a relationship that you're going to build over time.

2. Ask yourself if she is someone you would feel comfortable introducing to your mother.

You need to be able to connect with this person for at least the next nine months or even more if you choose to have that person in your life even after the birth of the child. If you're embarrassed about this person, it will come out over time.

3. Do you want someone experienced or non-experienced?

There are experienced and non-experienced surrogates. Experienced surrogates are going to cost more than inexperienced. If you do not use an agency, you should expect to spend approximately $25,000-$35,000 for an experienced surrogate. You can expect to spend between $10,000 and $20,000 for the inexperienced surrogate. Those are surrogate fees that you would pay them to carry this child for you.

This is another area that's different from adoption. In most states, it is legal to hire a woman to carry a child, and you can pay a fee for that. With adoption, you cannot pay a person who is pregnant when you plan to adopt their child. You cannot pay them to finish carrying that child through the adoption process.

If the surrogate has her own insurance, you should expect to pay more for her services than for a surrogate who does not have her own insurance. If the surrogate does not have insurance and you cannot get insurance for her for whatever reason, understand that Medicaid, which is a state and federal program to help pay for the cost of medical care for people who are indigent, is not an option. The surrogate cannot get her medical care covered through Medicaid because that is a federal crime.

Many surrogates that you interview may tell you that they're on Medicaid and that the procedure will be covered by it, but understand that is not an option when the pregnancy is due to a deliberate arrangement, such as surrogacy.

Those are the three things we would encourage you to look for in a surrogate:

1. Someone who has her own children

2. The relationship potential

3. Determine if you want someone who's experienced or who is doing this for the first time.

Surrogates Look At You Too

It's also important to understand what surrogates look for in the intended parents. While it's very personal to the surrogate, there are some commonalities that surrogates look for. One thing is that they're looking for couples that can never have their own babies.

Gay men, without a female, can never have their own baby and that's one reason why they're the most popular among adoption birth mothers and also among surrogates. When a surrogate says she's looking for Christian couples, it's usually her not so subtle way of saying that she wants heterosexual couples. Some may be okay with single females, but not gay individuals.

Many of them want to be seen as an extended family member even after the child is born. They're very offended if they feel as if this is a business transaction instead of a personal transaction. While it is a business transaction and you do have a contract, it's very important that the feelings go deeper than the ink on paper to them. They want to see couples that seem to love each other and enjoy each other's company. Certainly, they would want to see a couple that can afford to pay not only their fees, but provide for the child.

Even though a gestational carrier has no biological connection to the child, the surrogates are still very interested to know that this child is going to be in a good home with good parents. They don't want to carry a child for a couple that doesn't seem to be in love and is not going to provide well for the child.

Why Do They Choose To Be a Surrogate?

There are many reasons why women serve as surrogates.

1. **The common reason tends to be that they truly have altruistic intentions to help other people.**

Our surrogate said she wanted to help another couple because becoming pregnant and carrying children was so easy for her and she understood that is wasn't for so many other couples and she wanted to be able to help.

2. Others want to make their own way.

They want to be able to create a life for themselves and their children. You may have a single woman who is trying to get ahead and make a better life for herself. We feel that is what our surrogate was trying to do in that she had two young boys and had just ended a seven-year relationship with their father. She lived in a small town and we felt she wanted to get out of there and create a new life for herself. This was her way to do so while still being able to stay home with her children and raise them the way she wanted them to be raised.

3.`Certainly money is a motivation for some surrogates.

If they're getting paid $30,000, they can do that once per year and make more than someone can, working minimum wage at a supermarket. Money can be a motivation. It's not a lot but it's still something and something that they can not only be paid for but feel satisfied for helping a couple at the same time. Even if you made that same amount working minimum wage at a job, you may not feel the same satisfaction for doing so.

Recognizing some of these factors can help you understand or build the rapport with a surrogate and see it as more than just a business transaction. We need to realize, understand and truly feel that they have something that we don't have. We need to be happy that they're willing to help us regardless of the reason.

The bottom line is it doesn't matter why they're choosing to do it. We, as people who want to create our families, should just be thankful that there are people who can help us.

Matching with a Surrogate: What to Consider Before

The laws don't define the relationship we will have with our surrogate. The way we define it is through contracts so we are protected through contract law. Understand that the relationship is going to last at least nine months or more and you want to determine how often you're going to communicate with her.

Do you want to be friends with each other? Are you part of each other's support system or not? Will it be more of a business transaction? Do you want to live close to the surrogate or have the surrogate live close to you?

Recognize that while you're going through this process your family and friends will still call it adoption no matter how many times you tell them that it's not. It's very different so just understand while this is a real option people can and should consider when creating their families, it's still something that not a lot of people know about or understand. You may find that your support system is not as understanding or supportive as it would have been through some of the other processes.

Plus, if you go through every single option like we did, by the time you get to this, your support system might be tired. Just recognize that, as well.

What to Include In a Surrogacy Contract

With regard to the contracts, you must put your contract in writing. A contract that's verbal is not something that will ever hold up in the event that someone breaches the contract. Unfortunately, both sides of the relationship can and do breach contracts in this nature especially for people who are intended parents who are not committed to this method of creating their family.

After you've defined the relationship, create the contract. The contract should spell out what the compensation to the surrogate for carrying the child is, and what incidentals you are willing to pay for.

For example, it could be travel expenses and/or babysitting expenses for when the surrogate goes to her doctor's appointments. If the surrogate has to be on bed rest due to the pregnancy, are you willing to pay for a housekeeper to maintain the house, a babysitter to watch the kids while she's on bed rest and a clothing allowance because a pregnant woman is going to need new clothes throughout the pregnancy?

Which doctor is the surrogate going to use and where is the surrogate going to deliver—not only what state, but also what hospital? What do you do in the event of multiples? The decision would be do you birth all of the prospective children? Do you use selective reduction procedures? Who makes those decisions—the surrogate or the intended parents?

Arbitration, a lawsuit or mediation will have to happen if you disagree on something after you're already in the process and specifically after the pregnancy is successful. Recognize that very few laws protect you as the intended parents.

Know Which States Allow Surrogacy

Some states directly outlaw surrogacy—know which ones they are. For example, Michigan does not allow surrogacy at all. Some states expressly permit it, but most just don't have laws relative to surrogacy at all, and that's when it falls under contract law.

Seek advice from a lawyer. Jennifer and I are both lawyers and we understood that we didn't do this type of law, so we had to hire lawyers. It is so worth it when there are issues, but even when there are no issues you want to make sure everything is covered.

There needs to be a different lawyer for the intended parents and the surrogate. The lawyers should be experienced with surrogacy issues. The intended parents are going to be the ones who pay for both lawyers. You need to have the lawyers draft the contracts. We understand that there are sample contract online. We do not encourage the use of on-line contracts. They may be helpful to get an idea as to what types of information you want to consider including when your lawyer is drafting the contract, but we would not recommend using an on-line sample contract without the review of a lawyer who specializes in surrogacy and knows your particular situation.

When we reviewed sample contracts, they all had to do with heterosexual, married couples. There are many couples creating families who don't fall into that category. You'll also need the lawyers later in the process for other issues prior to the birth.

In many states, they allow you to obtain what is called a pre birth order, which means that a judge, prior to the birth, signs an order saying that the child is the intended parent's child as soon as the birth occurs, which means that the surrogate cannot claim that that person is the parent upon birth.

In many states, with same sex couples only one parent becomes the parent upon birth and the second one must petition for a second-parent adoption. You'll need a lawyer for that process. It's good to get the lawyer from the beginning so they can prepare all of this paperwork and be sure to file everything at the right time and make the transition smooth.

Getting to Baby: Surrogacy Story

In the last year or two, there was a gay couple that hired a surrogate in the state of Michigan and she seemed to have met all the criteria. She had apparently been a surrogate in the past, she had her own children, all boys, and she was married with a husband who was supportive of her being a surrogate.

From reading the surrogate mother message board, it is our understanding that the couple asked the surrogate if they needed a contract, and she said no. (An important note here; parties should not be asking each other for legal advice, that should come from a legal advisor who is independent.) When she gave birth to the child it was a baby girl. She and her husband had wanted a baby girl for a long time.

She was a traditional surrogate; she used her own egg, therefore, she was the legal mother of that child. She decided to parent that child and did not give the child to the couple. It created a national awareness of the negative aspects of surrogacy. This particular surrogate has been on Dr. Phil multiple times explaining her situation.

You don't see the gay men who are, some would say, the victims of this situation on any TV shows talking about it. Now, who's to blame here? I don't know that blaming anyone is important but what is important is this situation could have been avoided. Had the intended parents sought legal advice, had they chosen a surrogate in a state where surrogacy was legal (it is not legal in Michigan), and had they used a gestational carrier instead of a traditional surrogate, they would likely have their baby.

Decide on a Medical Plan

Another thing to think about is a medical plan. Decide whose sperm and egg is going to be used. If using donor eggs, will you use frozen or fresh eggs? Jennifer and I used donor eggs. We had to answer that question. After learning the difference between the frozen egg process and the fresh egg process when buying the eggs, we chose frozen eggs because it saved time and money.

The frozen eggs were already in the egg bank at the fertility clinic we planned to use for the IVF procedure. We did not have to wait for a woman to harvest her eggs and sync up her cycle with our surrogate who would have to take medication at the same time that the egg donor was taking medication. The frozen eggs were already available.

When you buy frozen eggs, you can choose to just buy a portion of what's available from one particular donor. That is what is called a shared cycle so more than one person can buy the same lot of eggs, whereas, if you use a fresh cycle you are paying for that egg donor to produce that cycle for you. The cost for fresh donor eggs is about twice as much as frozen eggs.

There has been a study, although it's not significantly positive, that tends to indicate that frozen eggs have more success at pregnancy than fresh eggs. The reason appears to be the thawing out process helps stimulate sperm activity levels.

You'll want to meet with a fertility clinic and ask them about those issues and what the studies indicate so you can make an informed and educated decision. You also want to determine what processes they use, what their success rate is and how often they assist with surrogate situations. That way you would know if they understand all the different issues involved with working with a couple who is using a surrogate.

You also have to get a psychological evaluation, which is required by the fertility clinic before they will move forward with you. Not only do the intended parents have to get the psychological evaluation, but the surrogate does as well.

It's important to support the surrogate through all the fertility drugs and treatment. The surrogate is going to be taking a lot of hormonal-type drugs, which can cause unpredictable emotions. If you are able to have a relationship with the surrogate, whether you're doing the informal process or going through an agency, just understand that part of your role as an intended parent is to support that surrogate through what she is going through to create this child for you. The surrogate's desires and actions may differ from your own.

Like every other couple after an IVF transfer or AI, you wait to find out if you're pregnant. This waiting period is something you want to discuss with your surrogate. Women can take pregnancy tests purchased at the grocery store. Fertility clinics suggest that you do not do that. Pregnancy tests can be wrong and that increases the risk of getting excited and then let down.

We did not want to know whether we were pregnant until we went back to our fertility clinic and they could tell us positively through the blood test. We were very clear to tell our surrogate that is what our desire was. Our surrogate, on the other hand, got a pregnancy test three days after the IVF procedure and used them twice a day every day until we had our doctor's appointment. She didn't tell us, thank goodness, because she was respecting our wishes.

After we found out we were pregnant, she told us she had been using pregnancy tests all along and she had saved all of the pee sticks in a bag for us in case we wanted them. We did.

Decide On a Birth Plan

Many couples who get pregnant don't decide on their birth plan until well into the process. There are three of you involved now and you may have very different views on what your birth plan is. Will you, as the intended parents participate in the labor and delivery? Acknowledge that birth plans can change and flexibility is important based on the situation of the pregnancy.

Getting to Baby: Surrogacy Story

We live in the big metropolitan area of Atlanta. There is a lot available to us here. Our surrogate was from a small town in Georgia where it's very rural and there aren't a lot of options. When she had her two children, she was strapped to the bed and made to lie there until the children were born once she went into labor.

When she moved to Atlanta, she was very wide-eyed like a child in a candy store and wanted to look at all of the options. She wanted to have a Doula, which is a person who is a labor coach who helps you at home. The Doula was talking to her about having a home birth in the water. She also discussed having a midwife. Midwives are nurses who help deliver the child in a hospital but without the assistance of a physician or an OBGYN. Then of course, there is the OBGYN option, which is what many people choose.

We wanted to respect her wishes but we also wanted our own plan. While these methods that she wanted, the Doula and midwife, sounded neat, they also sounded more high risk than being in a traditional hospital with a doctor around.

We wanted to ensure that this child would be born in a secure environment. That was different than what our surrogate wanted so those were the kinds of issues that we needed to not only discuss but put in the contract, as well. Even though we finally decided she could have a Doula, we were not having a home birth, especially when we found out we were pregnant with twins, which can be very complicated.

Then we decided we would use the midwife option. Having twins makes the pregnancy a little high risk, but our pregnancy became extremely high risk at a certain point. The midwife explained that she could not help when it reached that point.

The midwife is attached to a doctor but it's not a doctor we had ever met or really wanted to meet. At one point, we were floundering for a doctor that we wanted to use. Ultimately with our process, we ended up with a doctor we really wanted, at a hospital we never intended to be at. Be flexible but definitely talk about these things along the way because it can avoid potentially stressful situations.

We were open with our communications along the way and had agreed to things and were compromising. Those couples that assume how it's going to be and don't talk to their surrogate about it or vice versa can be in for a real shock as to what everybody's ideas are.

Protecting the Surrogates Feelings
• •

There are three of you in this particular relationship, not just two of you. Always be sensitive to the feelings of the surrogate. She's a person; she's involved in this process and she's doing something wonderful for you as a couple.

If she does not get pregnant upon the transfer or artificial insemination, she may feel like she has failed you. She may be worried that you're going to be mad at her because she didn't get pregnant and may even worry that you will choose another surrogate.

Just like we may not be getting pregnant for many reasons, the same things can happen with a surrogate. We have to realize that while they are stepping in to help us, that doesn't automatically mean they're going to get pregnant. Be very sensitive to not only your own feelings of that disappointment, but also the surrogate's.

Encourage the surrogate to join surrogate-networking groups online with other surrogates who are going through the process at the same time she is. It's important to recognize that she needs people who understand what she is going through and you, as the intended parents, can't help her with that. You're not going through what she is going through.

You have different desires and different goals and at some point, conflicting desires. She needs to know who's out there whom she can use as her support system. You're never going to understand what she is going through.

When the surrogate gets pregnant, remember her joys as well as your joys, meaning you're extremely excited that now you're going to have the baby that you've wanted for years, but also understand that she is happy for you too. She's been able to create for you what you couldn't create for yourself. She's very happy.

That may be a time to give her a gift of your thanks even though you don't know that the pregnancy is going to go full term. What you do know is she's done something incredible up to that point, and she needs to be part of the celebration. Be sensitive to how her body, emotions and her feelings may change throughout the whole process.

Be aware that the female intended parent could get jealous of the surrogate because the surrogate can get pregnant, whereas the woman in the relationship can't. That may produce other relationship issues between the surrogate and the couple. This can happen with a heterosexual as well as lesbian couple. It also may produce relationship issues between the female and their partner because the female may start feeling again a resurgence of inadequacy, which can turn into jealousy.

Leading up to the birth and after the birth, while the surrogate may be very happy for what she's created for you, she can be very sad at the same time. This is a process; it's taken a long time and she's developed a relationship with you. She's going to be wondering what the ongoing relationship will be from after the birth.

She may have biologically bonded with the child, and I don't mean because it's her eggs, but because she's felt that child kicking inside of her and moving. She's seen the ultrasound where she sees the child on the screen inside of her. She may go through post partum depression. Through all of that, she's just performed the most amazing task for you so we've got to understand, realize and still be supportive of her emotions—the ones she can and the one she can't control. Treat her very well.

When we had our children, we had a very difficult pregnancy. We could not have been more thankful for everything that our surrogate went through.

It's our belief that any woman who has a child, whether it's her own child or a child for someone else, needs to be pampered and taken well care of and should receive a gift on the day that they've given birth. In our situation, we wanted to do something more than just a gift. Even then, I don't think there is a gift that's good enough for what this person has done for us, for the creation they've made for us.

Our surrogate had been on bed rest since week 20 of the pregnancy and her two small children were being taken care of by their aunt who had moved into their home. Our surrogate was actually in the hospital for five of those weeks on bed rest so she did not get to see her children as much as she would have liked.

On the day of her hospital discharge after delivering our children, we arranged for a stretch limousine to pick up her children and her sister and then bring the limousine to the hospital to pick her up and take her home. We didn't tell her of our plans.

When it was time for discharge, we packed everything up and I told her I was going down to get the car. She was wheeled out in the wheelchair as people are after they've given birth, and there was that big, stretch limousine out in the front of the hospital. I started wheeling her up to the limousine and she asked, "What is this?" I said, "This is for you." She was in a daze until she looked inside and her two children were there sitting in their car seats, and she started crying.

I knew there was nothing else we could have done more for her than what was most important to her and that was her children greeting her and taking her home. So, think about your surrogate and what special thing you can do for her because, at that moment, it really should be about her even though you have your family now.

After that moment, you may have continued contact or you may have decided you don't want a continuing relationship. This is something that should have been decided together. Realize that the surrogate does care how you raise your children so she may want ongoing pictures of them, letters, and telephone calls with you.

Know that over time that relationship can become stronger and stronger, and you can be friends or extended family members, or it may also wane and you have less and less contact. That is the way relationships in life go, and surrogates are no different. It's just that they were a part of your life at this moment and you will both define how that will go in the future.

Surrogacy Facts

Surrogacy is a creation of your family. It's an option that traditional society doesn't know about, hasn't considered, and doesn't seem to be promoted well.

It's interesting though because everyone seems to be interested in what celebrities do and it's cool to hear about the celebrities who have gone through surrogacy. What has emerged in the past couple of years are all of these celebrities who are using surrogacy as their option instead of adoption.

For example, Joan Lunden, formerly of Good Morning America, had two sets of twins through surrogacy. In 2003, she had one set and in 2005 she had another. She was quoted in People Magazine in the year 2003, and she's a contributor to the *Chicken Soup for the Soul Thanks Mom Edition* published in 2010. She was also on Larry King – she's a pioneer of surrogacy.

Cindy Margolis also has twin girls through surrogacy. She had her girls in 2005 and is the national spokesperson for a non-profit organization called Resolve, which is a national infertility association.

Here are a few of the most widely well-known people who have used surrogacy in the past few years:

Sarah Jessica Parker and Matthew Broderick had twin girls in 2009. Kelsey Grammer, (TV's Frasier), went through surrogacy three times. Dennis Quaid, another great actor had a twin girl and boy in 2007.

Robert DeNiro, had twin sons through surrogacy in 1995. Dancing with the Stars celebrity Marissa Jaret Winokur used surrogacy. Ricky Martin had twin boys in 2008. Sir Elton John and his partner had a son on Christmas Day, 2010 through a surrogate. The list goes on and on with regard to celebrities using surrogates.

What I think is also interesting is that surrogacy is a process that tends to attract couples who have higher financial means available to them than people who adopt children. That may be another reason why surrogacy hasn't been explored a lot because it's perceived as expensive and only celebrities are among those who are using surrogacy. It's rare to hear about your every day person in society using this method of having children.

Hopefully, through this book and this sharing of information, people can learn that they can create their family this way if they choose, for example, the informal process of surrogacy and not use an agency. You don't have to spend tens of thousands of dollars to create your family through surrogacy. Certainly, that is what is most familiar when you see celebrities or when you do research on the agencies that help with surrogacy.

Surrogacy Checklist

When exploring surrogacy there is a checklist you might want to go through. First, with every process, no matter what it is, self-reflection is very important.

1. You need to recognize and ask yourself, are you a jealous person?

If you are a jealous person and are going to use a surrogate, you may want to consider using one in another state so that you're not jealous of the pregnancy or the fact that the surrogate can get pregnant when you can't. You can't be jealous of the surrogate talking to your husband, if that's an issue. Even with gay couples, a surrogate can develop a closer relationship with one person in the party more so than the other person, which can create some jealousy. "Why are you always talking with her? She doesn't talk to me." Those can be issues.

If you can recognize that and patterns of your relationships in the past, choose a surrogate that's in another state or go through an agency where they don't allow you to build a relationship.

2. Do you want to be involved in all the doctor's appointments or the majority of them?

If so, you'll need to either, be flexible with your travel plans and have a travel budget or you'll want to use a surrogate that's close to you geographically, willing to move to where you are or you're willing to move to where they are.

3. Are you comfortable just winging the process and learning it as you go?

If so, do not use a surrogacy agency because you can accomplish everything you need through the informal process of finding your own surrogate, generally online. That's the fastest way to do it. You can use an attorney who can draw up the contracts for you and who can line up a psychologist for you. In fact, the fertility clinic will give you a list of approved psychologists.

If you are comfortable forging your own way and have been through the information in this book, then I would not recommend using an agency. An agency will be a lot more expensive. If you're not comfortable, and you want that handholding and every step of the way choreographed for you, then definitely use an agency.

At a minimum, regardless of which choice you use, whether you do informal or an agency, you have to use an attorney experienced in assisted reproductive technology law. I would not approach this relationship without having the proper contracts in place, knowing what your legal rights are, and what the surrogate's legal rights are.

Action Steps That Can Be Taken Now
• •

The action steps that I recommend are:

1. **Go to the website, www.surromomsonline.com and review the ads of not just the surrogates that are looking for intended parents, but also look at the ads that the intended parents are sending out.**

You don't want your ad to look exactly like theirs and you certainly don't want to look like you're desperate, even if you feel like you are. Nobody wants to be with someone who's desperate. That's whether you're looking for a job, a relationship and partner and the same holds true for surrogates looking for intended parents. They don't want to feel like you chose them just because they were available. They want you to choose them because of what you have that binds the two of you together.

2. **Set a telephone conference with interested surrogates by responding to their ads via email first.**

When you set a telephone conference, it gives you a good idea about what her voice is like; you can ask questions and get a sense of her commitment before you commit to seeing her face to face, incurring travel expenses, time, and things like that. You'll also get a sense for her urgency as far as when she's ready to get pregnant. For example, a surrogate may have just finished having a child for another couple, but put themselves back out there on the website saying they want to be a surrogate again.

Their body needs time to heal and that's another thing to look at. If a surrogate just had a baby, and she says she's ready again right now, you may want to think twice about that because the body does need time to heal. You would want to talk to a doctor about how much time you should wait, but the doctors we consulted with said no less than six months but preferably 12 months before getting pregnant again. You'll find out what her sense of urgency is or lack thereof.

You may meet a surrogate that says she's in no rush, and is okay with whenever it happens. You'll also get a sense of her personality on the phone.

3. **Set up a face-to-face interview if you like her and seem to click over the phone.**

If you have a surrogate that is hesitant to meet you face to face, then we recommend you continue looking for other surrogates. You have to have a face-to-face meeting so that you know what this person is like in person. The phone can only get you so far.

Also, if you're going to do traditional surrogacy, you may want to know what the person looks like, what their family looks like and things like that, because the child is going to have their genetic make up.

4. **Talk about the types of contract terms that you both want. Have what you have in mind written down on paper so you can discuss it.**

The reason I say to have it written down is because when you're meeting for the first time, you're so nervous, excited; you're going to forget half of the stuff that you wanted to talk about. If you don't have it written down, you're going to leave that meeting wishing you had talked about certain things, and it's going to seem like you're adding new things to the contract or to the idea of the contract, which may seem unfair to the surrogate.

She may say, "Well, now you're asking for other things. If I had known that, it would have changed things." Come with your list of talking points.

5. Know what you're willing to pay.

If you know that this surrogate has never been a surrogate before, and they don't have their own insurance, the range is between $10,000 and $20,000. If you want to pay $15,000, know that and explain you are comfortable paying $15,000 for her fee. In addition to that, know that you are willing to pay (x) for housing and childcare per month; it's important to know what the expected expenses could be.

In our situation, we purchased a house for the surrogate to live in so we could maintain control over the housing expenses. We didn't want our surrogate to move into the Atlanta market, decide to rent a 3-bedroom apartment because she has two children and herself and spend anywhere from $1,200—$2,200 a month on an apartment, which is what that would be in our area.

Instead, we could purchase a house and not have any on-going maintenance expenses and limit our costs. Plus, we could later sell that house and recover all of the money we had put into it, which is the option we chose, and we were able to do that.

6. Begin the medical procedures as soon as possible.

You do not know what wrinkles may come up through the medical procedures. Buy the eggs and the sperm, whichever you need to acquire as soon as possible. Have them stored at the facility where you'll be doing your procedure, so the facility has them on hand.

At that point, everything is in place. Just relax, let it happen, develop your relationship with the surrogate, enjoy that relationship, continue to enjoy the relationship with your partner and go from there.

Creating Your Family in 12 Months or Less

The reason Jennifer and I enjoyed surrogacy so much and are such big promoters of it and state that you can create your family within

12 months or less is that we've been there, done that and we've gone through three different processes to create our family. From the moment we met our surrogate, Brittany, in May of 2009, to the birth of our children in March of 2010, it was 10 months.

If they were born on their due date which was May 5th of 2010, then we still would have been one week shy of 12 months from the day we met to the day we created our family, and we've got two beautiful, healthy children now because of surrogacy.

Throughout the entire pregnancy and the IVF process, aside from a few complications, we finally felt like we had some control over the situation. From our costs, the contract, selecting the best doctors, best procedures and getting acupuncture to relax and help with our body energy flow to the fact that our surrogate could not change her mind and pull a baby away from us.

When we were personally trying to get pregnant, we were doing "all the right things." For example, we even stopped drinking cold water and started drinking room temperature water because apparently that was supposed to be better for the chance of pregnancy. Still, even after all of that, we had no baby.

Through the adoption process, the prospective adoptive parents have no control at all; even through open adoption where you get to know who the birth mother is, and you get to select if you want that situation or not.

At the end of the day, you don't have any control. The agency is dictating your birth mother letter, and they won't approve you into the system until it is perfect in their mind. The birth mother or the agency gets to choose you. Then you either accept that selection or you don't. After being chosen, you walk on eggshells, hoping not to screw anything up along the way, especially with open adoption. You may have ongoing communication either through email, letters or telephone conversations or even seeing each other in person regularly where you have to be careful.

You're always thinking, "Did I say the right or wrong thing? Could I have laughed more? Did I show empathy, and did I care enough about her day when she complained how it went? Did I seem too eager? What if she changes her mind?" The whole situation is unpredictable. You just don't know.

Then, after the birth, let's assume that you get all the way to the birth. You're doing all you can to be sensitive and supportive to the birth mother and birth father, if he's around. You're very excited to be having this child, but also trying not to bond too much with the baby until the judge signs the papers. You've got all of these different emotions going on, none of which you can control. The birth mother is still in control until the judge signs those papers.

With surrogacy, it is totally different; it's much better for those who need to be in control. The Type A personalities just cannot go with the flow as hard as we try. Once you match with a surrogate, you have a contract in place and the contract controls. If you have any disagreement or dispute, the contract controls.

After she gets pregnant, assuming it's a gestational carrier and not a traditional carrier, she has no ability to change her mind with regard to who the legal parent of that child is. She can decide to abort the child but unless something has gone seriously wrong in your relationship, a surrogate is not going to go through the whole process of taking hormone prescriptions, going to the doctor all of that time to then just decide to abort the child.

The surrogate can run away and go to a place where you would never find her, but that is unlikely to happen because she's gone through a lot with you. It's a big decision to become a surrogate and when finances are considered, you haven't paid her everything in the beginning unless you got bad advice. So she's still going to need the financial support that you're going to be paying throughout the pregnancy.

We felt that once we were in that process, we were much more relaxed, and I can't emphasize enough how just being relaxed, releasing that tension can have positive results in your life whether it's pregnancy or any other areas.

CHAPTER 6
Expecting Multiples

"Too much of a good thing can be wonderful."—*Mae West*

It's important to know that there are increased risks of multiples with IVF, including surrogacy. Just look around at society and the celebrities mentioned earlier who have used surrogacy to create their families. It appears that people who use surrogacy use fertility treatments.

With fertility treatments as well as surrogacy, generally there are multiple embryos being transferred into the person who's going to carry the baby (babies).

Our doctors told us that when you transfer multiple embryos, you don't have a better chance at getting pregnant; you only have an increased risk of having multiples because you're transferring more embryos. Not only are you putting more embryos in, there is also the possibility that the embryos will split creating identical twins.

Jennifer and I wanted twins from the very beginning, so we knew we wanted to transfer two embryos. We wanted twins because we wanted two children. After having gone through the entire process, we only wanted to do this one time. Emotionally and financially we just could not afford to go through any other process again. We were really hoping for twins.

As I mentioned earlier in the book, Jennifer is a twin and we thought it would be wonderful for her to experience the process of having twins after having been one herself.

Many of the celebrities we looked at had twins and some of them are boy/girl combinations like ours, but many of them are not. It's important to know that when you go through fertility or surrogacy that if you're going to put multiple embryos in to increase the chances of successful pregnancy, you could have multiples. It could be twins, triplets or more.

Our doctor told us that we had 30% more chance for multiples than if they put one embryo in. Before you transfer the embryos, decide how many children you can manage emotionally, financially and logistically.

Jennifer has said that while she was a prosecutor for 15 years and handled some egregious cases of murder and child abuse and horrible victim crimes, that being a stay at home mother of twins is certainly the most challenging thing she has ever done mentally, as well as physically.

Logistically, is your house set up? Can you accommodate more than one child? Having multiples can create difficult pregnancies as well. That is something that has to be considered when considering how many embryos to transfer.

Difficult Decisions

Some of the difficult decisions come when you transfer multiple embryos and then you are determined to be having twins or more, three or four or eight children like the octomom that's been in the news in the past few years. You have to decide-Are you going to parent all of the children? Are you going to go to term with all of them or are you going to do selection reduction?

This means that you're deciding deliberately to terminate some of the embryos, which is a medical procedure where the doctor goes in and puts saline solution into the embryos to help them dissolve. It's a natural process that the body does on its own when we don't get pregnant, but this is doctor-assisted selection.

Twins
• • • • • •

Other issues to consider with multiples are that you could be in the adoption process and a situation may present itself when a birth mother says she's having twins. It's important to know that while you look around today and it seems like there are a lot of multiples, it's not as common as you would think.

Certainly, without the assistance of fertility treatment, we wouldn't be seeing it near as much as we do today. When a birth mother says that she is pregnant with twins, just know that is rare. It does happen, but it may be the sign of a potential scam.

Scammers know that parents who have been trying to have children for a while, who would do anything to have children would jump at the chance to have twins. The perception is that you're getting two babies for the price of one through the adoption. Walk cautiously when you're going through the adoption route if a birth mother presents with twins.

Also with twins and the adoption route, there is a high risk of the birth mother changing her mind. Some reasons for that can be that while the birth mother may on a cognitive level understand that they can't take care of one child, much less two, oftentimes, twins are premature and need medical care. The motherly instinct kicks in and the birth mother wants to ensure that those babies are taken care of and getting the proper healthcare.

They just can't seem to pull themselves away from the hospital when their babies are in the neonatal intensive care unit (NICU), and they're hooked up to the ventilator or feeding tube. There is a higher risk of the birth mother changing her mind when the babies are premature and in the NICU.

Other things to consider with multiples, like with our pregnancy, are that it is a higher risk pregnancy. Even people who have had very non-eventful, healthy pregnancies can develop issues like our surrogate who had to have a cerclage procedure because her cervix became weak due to the pressure of the two babies. A cerclage is surgical procedure wherein the cervix is tied shut to prevent premature labor and delivery.

High blood pressure, preeclampsia and other risk factors increase because of multiples pregnancies. That is something that a couple needs to talk about in advance, especially if they're going to be using a surrogate. Those are issues that would need to be discussed with the surrogate, as well.

Multiple Birth Facts

Multiple pregnancies are almost always born prior to 38 weeks of gestation, which is the average length of pregnancy. Thirty-six weeks is average for twin births, 32 weeks for triplets and 30 weeks for quadruplets.

It is close to impossible to tell a couple with 100% certainty that they will or will not have multiples if they go through IVF. I mentioned that our doctor gave us a 30% chance of multiples when we put two embryos in. So for people who are curious, that is the statistical chance.

Instances like octomom—the woman who had octuplets with the help of IVF back in 2009 are rare. The average patient who is coming in to a fertility clinic for IVF does not need to worry about something like that happening at all.

In summary, there are a number of alternative methods available to you. We've discussed IVF, Artificial Insemination, Adoption and Surrogacy and given you some tips to make the choice that feels right for you.

In this next section, we will be sharing our personal stories with each of these methods so that you see how each method played an integral role with us "getting to baby" and see the principles outlined previously in action! Important note: The stories below are not intended to "sway" you towards any one method. Their only purpose is for you to connect with us and what unfolded.

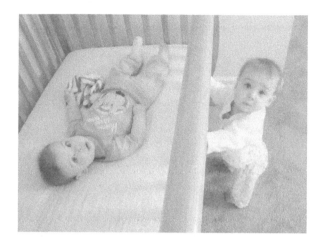

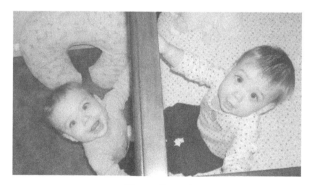

Two Cute!

GETTING TO Baby

Capturing the Experience through Pictures

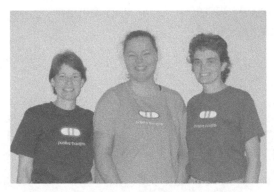

Victoria, Brittany, Jennifer on Embryo Transfer Day

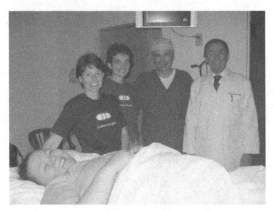

Transfer Day, Brittany, Victoria, Jennifer,
Dr. Peter Nagy, Dr. Hilton Kort

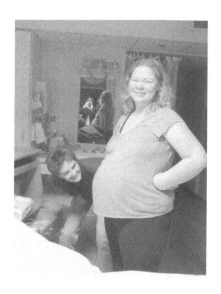

At the hospital while on bed rest

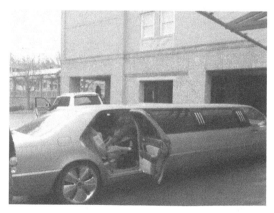

Brittany's ride home after delivery

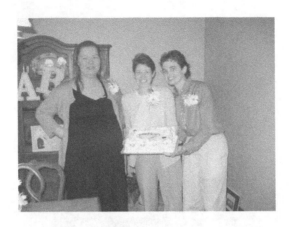

First Baby Shower—Two days before giving birth!

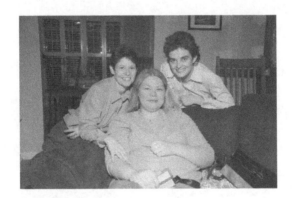

Second Baby Shower—After the birth!

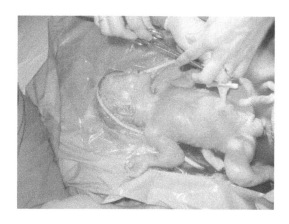

Jennifer cutting Christopher's cord

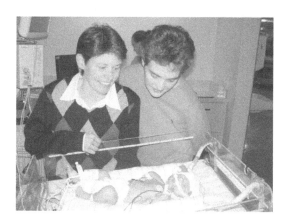

Christopher in the NICU

GETTING TO Baby

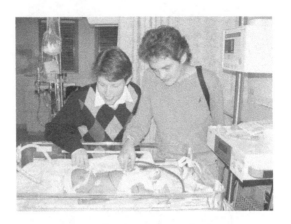

Katherine in the NICU

The Easter Bunny Brought
Our Babies Home on Easter Sunday 2010

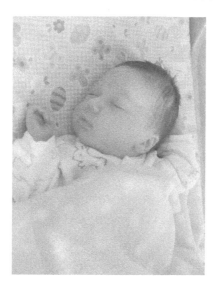

Katherine

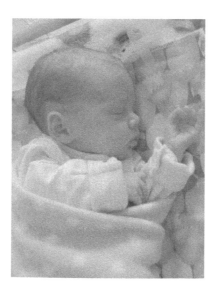

Christopher

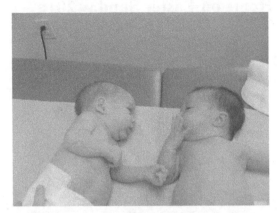

Discussing their first pediatrician
appointment and who will weigh more

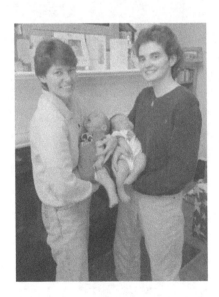

Our FIRST Mother's Day! ☺ ☺

Second Parent Adoption Hearing

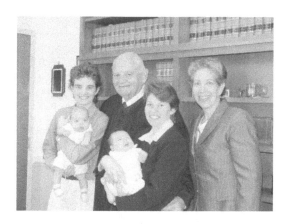

Jennifer, Christopher, Judge Clarence Seeliger,
Katherine, Victoria, and Attorney Barbara Katz

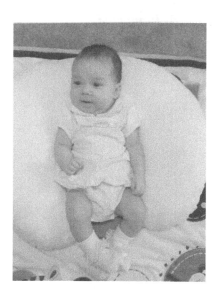 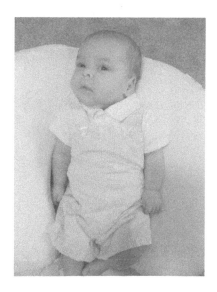

Katherine and Christopher in their
southern seersucker outfits for court

Four Generations!
••••••••••••••••••

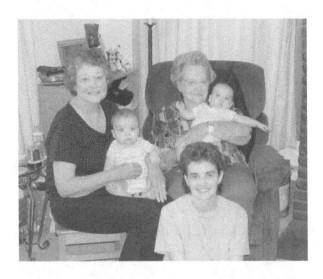

Great Grandma Dettmer with Katherine,
Grandma Betty Sue with Christopher, Mom

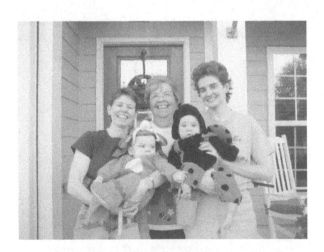

First Halloween with "Maw Maw" Collier
Christopher is a Monkey and Katherine is a Lady Bug

ADORABLE!!

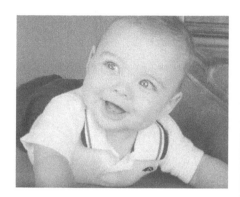
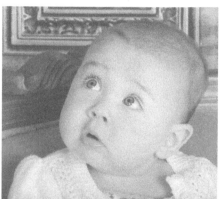

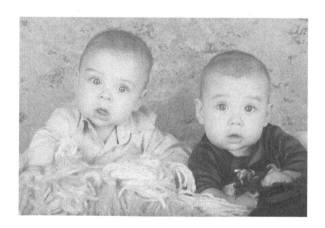

Six-Month Pictures

First Christmas 2010
• • • • • • • • • • • • • • • • • • • •

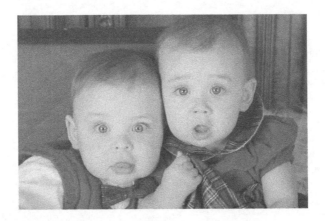

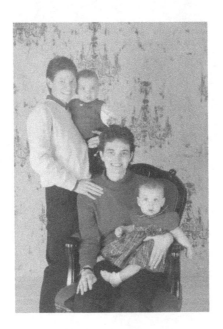

The Best Gifts Ever

CHAPTER 7

Our Personal Stories Using Alternative Methods and Lessons We'd like to Pass On To You

"Knowledge of what is possible is the beginning of happiness."
— George Santayana

Getting to Baby: Our Entire Story

Being in a same-sex relationship, we knew from the beginning that assistive reproductive technology was going to be necessary to create the family we wanted, so we looked at artificial insemination (AI). We did the research and spoke with several of our friends who had chosen AI. We also looked at IVF. Jennifer and I both like immediate results. We are extremely pragmatic, and being pragmatic can be very costly because of the choices you make to receive the results that you think will be the best.

What we've found through this whole process is that no matter what path you choose, even if you feel it's the best and all the research points to it as the best, the best doesn't guarantee success. We didn't know that in the beginning, but it is something we've learned through all the different processes we've gone through.

We chose IVF first. Before we started the procedure, we had to select the sperm.

We spoke briefly earlier about the process of doing this. We went to different sperm bank websites to look at profiles, which is another area in which we had to do a lot of research. In the city where we live, which is a bedroom community of Atlanta, there is a high concentration of lesbian couples that are having children using a local sperm bank. Due to that, there are a number of half-siblings in the same community. Therefore, we knew from doing our research that we wanted to use a sperm bank located outside Georgia. While we know that there's a possibility of having half-siblings, we didn't want them to live down the street from us.

Mr. Dreamy

We chose a sperm donor who on paper was just perfect, dreamy even. Tall, curly hair, green eyes and everything we wanted to combine our characteristics. Some sperm banks provide "staff impressions." Because the sperm donors go in regularly to do testing and to deposit their goods, the staff gets to see them regularly and gets to know them. Our sperm bank offered this option which we took advantage of. We called and got the staff impression of our first and second choices.

The woman who answered the phone was so funny. A number identifies each donor. We didn't know the person's name, but we said we'd like to get the staff impressions from them so we gave the donor's number. She said, "Oh my God, he is so good looking. He has the nicest personality." She went on and on and on. We asked for a staff impression of our second choice. She said, "He's okay, too." It was so different.

To do the IVF process of combining the eggs and sperm inside the lab and then transferring them to Jennifer for her to carry, there were some medical tests required. In the testing, it was determined that Jennifer, as a carrier, and the sperm of our perfect donor, were not compatible, so we couldn't use our first choice. Then, we went back to purchase our second choice, and it was no longer available because his sperm was all purchased. For some reason that I can't recall, we couldn't even use our third choice.

We got pregnant using our fourth choice for sperm. Jennifer previously worked with another woman whose partner used AI to get pregnant. They lived only one mile from our house and used the same OBGYN that we used. We were going through the process pretty much at the same time. One morning I was sitting at the OB's office talking with one of them, and we started to discuss the characteristics of our donors. The description of their donor sounded like an exact match of our back-up donor that we were not able to purchase. That donor also had a picture available of when he was a small child. After the birth of their son, when we saw him, we were convinced that their sperm donor was our back-up choice.

Even after we had done everything to stay away from the local sperm bank, we still potentially could have had a half-sibling if we had purchased our back-up choice. We are blessed with how our situation worked out.

Home Run!

In our city, we have several major assistive reproductive technology specialist practices. We did not have our OBGYN do the procedure for us. Instead, we went to a reproductive specialist that's very well known nationally. Jennifer and I both started our medications. I was harvesting my eggs, and her lining was becoming plump and ready to receive. We then went in for the procedure. It's very exciting. Everybody's excited for you; the nurses are there to help you, and they prep you the night before. We went in for our procedure and were extremely lucky. We got a home run on our first pitch and got pregnant!

We only had one egg that I harvested that was fertilized. During our first try, I produced eight eggs, while some women produce 20 to 40 eggs. We have a friend who harvested her eggs for IVF, and she produced 40 eggs. When I got eight, I was disappointed. Then, when there was only one fertilized, that was our one and only shot. They transferred the fertilized egg into Jennifer.

We found out relatively quickly that we were pregnant. Everything was going well. Jennifer and I were both very healthy. We were doing everything that you're supposed to do from drinking lots of water, exercising, reducing stress in life and being excited. As you have ultrasounds, you have to decide if want to know the gender of the child. Jennifer and I wanted to know.

We Were High-Risk

Also, we would have been 36 years old by the time the child would have been born so we were considered high risk. Once you're pregnant, the reproductive specialist transfers the on-going treatment and monitoring of the pregnancy to your OBGYN. Our OBGYN told us we were high risk, solely based upon being over age 35. They advised us of the tests we could do to determine whether we were at risk of having a child with disabilities, such as Down syndrome.

This is where our pragmatism can sometimes not be the best. We decided we wanted to know if that was a possibility for a couple different reasons.

1. We would need to determine if we wanted to terminate the pregnancy if there was a severe abnormality.

2. If there was a disability, we would want to line up the proper doctors and medical treatments or resources we would need when we gave birth, doing our research while we had the time and weren't overly emotional about it.

We determined what the gender was. We found out we were having a baby girl. While we had said from the beginning that we didn't know which gender we wanted because we wanted both, we were ecstatic to be having a baby girl. We didn't think to ourselves, "It's not twins, it's only one." We were just happy to know we were going to have our baby.

To Have an Amniocentesis or Not?

We had the perfect name picked out. We both loved it, not to mention that Jennifer has a friend she told about the name we picked out which was Katherine Elizabeth. Her friend told her it was the perfect name and that she had picked that name out also, but her husband didn't agree so she didn't get to name her child that. The pregnancy was going along fine. Beginning at 16 weeks you can decide whether or not you're going to have an amniocentesis, which is an invasive procedure to determine if there are any genetic abnormalities.

We decided to have the amniocentesis so that we could make future choices and plans, if necessary. We had the procedure at 16 weeks of pregnancy.

The day after the amniocentesis Jennifer was at work, and she called me. I too was at work and didn't get the first phone call. She called because she had some water leakage, not a large amount but certainly something to be concerned about. About two hours later there was more leakage. There was no ambiguity as to what was going on – her sac had broken. She called me again after she had called the doctor and was instructed to go to the hospital. I picked Jennifer up and we went to the hospital as instructed. While at the hospital, Jennifer had an ultrasound and everything looked fine. There was sufficient fluid in the sac and the baby was moving around quite a bit. She was very cute. We had a follow up appointment with a maternal fetal medical (MFM) specialist the next morning who ordered Jennifer to be on bed rest for a week. The hope was that the sac would repair itself.

After about three days, we both knew what the result was going to be. It's something that, even in the best relationships, sometimes there's just nothing you can do to make the situation better or make each other feel better. Nevertheless, Jennifer stayed on bed rest for a week.

Something was Different This Time

After the week was over, we went back to the MFM, but this time the ultrasound was very different. It looked like something was wrong. There was no water in the uterus, yet you could see the skeleton of the baby lying at the bottom. The physician didn't have much facial expression, nor did she communicate with us at all. It didn't take a physician to know what we were seeing. At this point, we couldn't even look at each other, and there were no words.

It was another moment of a learning experience that you cannot prepare for in advance and that no one thinks to tell you could happen in advance. The risk of the sac breaking due to an amniocentesis is so small. You never think you are going to be the statistic.

We were told to go back to our OB's office. We left and went to the doctor's office and talked to the doctor who was sitting behind her desk. This is a practice with multiple OBGYN's, so because of that and the fact that they never know who's going to be on-call during deliveries, you have to see all of them throughout the pregnancy, so you get familiar with everybody. When we went in for our amniocentesis, the doctor was someone we had never met before, but we knew of her. If there was ever a moment when you should trust your gut, it's when you're having a procedure that you don't know a lot about.

When we went to get the amniocentesis, we walked in, and I had a gut feeling that it wasn't right and we shouldn't be doing it. Not that we shouldn't be doing the amniocentesis, but that we should not be doing it that day with that doctor. I kept my mouth shut, and I can't ever erase that. It's not that I blame the doctor, but I blame myself for not trusting my gut and saying we should reschedule and that it wasn't right that day.

So, as we met with yet another doctor back at the OB's office, she sat behind her desk and bluntly said, "You can't control everything." That is absolutely correct and that is one of the biggest issues that couples who are trying to have children, deal and struggle with, is the lack of control over the process of getting pregnant, the lack of control over the process of adoption and the lack of control of just having a child.

What are Our Options?

When she said that, we were in our most raw state. We didn't know what else to say or do so I looked at her and just said, "What are our options?" She told us we could induce the child and go through labor to birth the child or that we could have a D&C, which is like an abortion procedure or can wait and pass the fetus. The risk with waiting is that it may not all come out and you can get an infection in your uterus, which can cause much more damage to you. The risk with the D&C is that it's a surgical procedure that can cause scaring, which can then prevent further pregnancies.

So to us, the only option that seemed viable was to induce and go through labor and get it over with as quickly as possible. The doctor told us to go have lunch and be at the hospital at 3:00 p.m., and that's what we did. We went to our favorite standby restaurant close to the doctor's office and ordered lunch. We didn't eat a bite and didn't really say anything to each other, because what could we say?

Our minds were just numb; they were probably hoping that we had better preparation or understanding as to what could have happened. Jennifer and I were in our own individual black holes. Even in the closest relationship, there's no amount of holding each other, no amount of talking or anything you can say that would make either of you feel better. Who is to be consoled? Both of you. So, it is what it is.

It's important that before you're in bliss, before you would want to know or even think about it, there are things that should be thought about. You need to at least have knowledge if not outright prepare for the worst.

We went to lunch and then went home and packed a bag of clothing because we knew we would be at the hospital all night.

We then went to the hospital, which was a learning experience for us. We were told by our doctor to go to the fourth floor, which is where they have the high-risk pregnancies between week 20 and 24, because that's pre-term labor. If you have a child during those weeks, it's highly likely that the child will not survive.

When we got there, we had to argue with the intake nurse that we were on the right floor. She asked how long have Jennifer had been pregnant. When we said 17 weeks, she told us we were on the wrong floor even though this is where we were told to go. Mind you, we were going through hell, yet, we have to argue with this woman that we are indeed on the right floor. Finally, she tells us to sit down. We did and ultimately, we got a room.

The Waiting Game

After finally being admitted, Jennifer had been administered some medication around 3:00 p.m. that would induce labor. When you induce labor, it creates the labor pains and becomes very painful. She wasn't in any pain for a long time. She was under the influence of medication, and I felt like I should be the one to call the family members to let them know because we had already told the world of our joy. We were beyond the 12th week, so all of our family, friends and co-workers knew. I called her family and my family from the room and let everyone know.

We waited and waited. Around 2:00 a.m., Jennifer started having some very strong labor pains. I was out in the hallway telling them we needed some pain medication. Of course, they took their sweet time, which is no different than just about any other experience at a hospital.

You're there to be treated and have to beg for them to do their jobs. Finally, Jennifer got some pain medication and became really loopy, she could still feel the contractions they just weren't as bad, and still fairly non-emotional.

I wasn't under the influence of any medication; however, so I was aware of everything that was going on. I was acutely feeling everything in the environment, so at one moment Jennifer said she felt pressure down in her pelvic area. I looked down there and could see the head of the child coming through. I went into the hallway and called for help.

By the way, this is the wing where there are a bunch of pre-term birth possibilities, so throughout that previous day from 3:00 p.m. until the next day when we were released, we were hearing women crying who were inconsolable and some babies crying, which is a healthy and welcoming sign.

One of the OB's from our practice came in and delivered the child. I was standing by Jennifer's side the whole time. Jennifer was very groggy and could not keep her eyes open.

It's All in Pieces

There was a physician's assistant in with us. After our child and placenta came out, the doctor said that everything was out and said, "We're clear here." There are certain things in our lives that we will always have imprinted in our minds. The nurse asked, "Should I clean it up?" I'm not sure if she knew the gender of our baby. The doctor said, "I'm not sure it's in a condition where you can. It's all in pieces."

They were talking about our "baby".

I was right there, as was Jennifer. They go away, and we are sitting near each other holding hands when in comes the bereavement nurse. Again, something we didn't expect, certainly something we should have expected but I guess we weren't thinking about it. She came in and was wonderful and very necessary, but she started presenting us with choices that again we had no idea we would have to make on the spot, and that was, "Do you want this child to be cremated or buried? Have you thought about where you want the services to take place? Do you want a funeral service?"

These are all the things you would need to ask for a person who has died. But, we were presented with this package of stuff and told to look it over, because they needed to know how to discard the child. We looked at everything. Jennifer and I, we both want to be cremated, so we thought we would do the same for our child. In our city, there happened to be a funeral home that did that for free for situations just like this. They also scatter the ashes in a garden at a particular cemetery, which we felt was a nice thing for them to do.

We thought that would be a nice way for us to have our child taken care of. So, we made the decision and then the bereavement nurse told us that our child was able to be cleaned and that they had taken little footprints and handprints from her. They had taken pictures of her with a little measuring tape next to her. They put her in a blanket and she showed us all of these little artifacts and asked if we wanted to see her to say goodbye.

I didn't think I could. Jennifer was still sedated, so I made the decision and decided I couldn't do it. Jennifer had to stay in the hospital long enough to make sure she didn't get a fever or infection and so the mediations could wear off. This caused us to be there until the afternoon of the next day. We were both so ready to go home at that point and get out of that place — not just the physical place but the emotional place, as well.

Jennifer put on her clothes and we had the release from the physician that we could go home. They had to bring Jennifer a wheelchair. We stood up to leave, and I just lost it. I started crying uncontrollably and told them I had to see my baby. She was in one of those glass incubators that preemies are kept in. They wheeled her into the room and the bereavement nurse picked her up and started to hand her to Jennifer. She still wasn't feeling quite steady because of the medication, so they handed her to me.

She wasn't even a pound and her skin was so thin that you could see through it. She had been in the uterus without water for a week and her skin was starting to decompose. There are aromas that go with placenta and babies, and all the smells, sights and emotions were coming up.

Saying Goodbye

We said our goodbyes. A hospital is an interesting place. As I was walking down the hallway to leave while Jennifer was being pushed in a wheelchair, I was trying not to make eye contact with anyone. You have people like us who are crying and then you have other people who are actually having babies who are excited. You don't want them to feel bad for you or to dampen their bright moment. And, you don't want to share *your* moment, as bad as it is, with anyone else because it's yours. Leaving the hospital without our baby was just wrong. While it did not turn out the way we wanted it to, we certainly bonded through it. It's something that has made up a part of who we are as individuals, and it's something I will always hold dear to me, as I will that child.

I actually named that child. It wasn't our perfect name; I renamed her so that when I go to the cemetery and visit, I have an identity to go with her. That's something, while I would not want to go through again, I survived. It's a moment, a situation and a circumstance that I'll always remember.

Everything That Seems Certain Changes

After having that experience, as an individual and as a couple, you start to question, re-evaluate and analyze your philosophy on life, death.

Everything you've known for certain changes, because you realize that there truly is no certainty. Taking the time to evaluate those important core values with regard to life, death and how you want to live yours is important, because you can then start to ask yourself whether you want to try again.

Before you can answer that question, you should take time to answer those other questions to see if your mindset has changed, about pregnancy, having children or each other. We asked ourselves if we should try again. We didn't have any eggs left. Many people who go through IVF have reserve eggs that are fertilized. When that is the case, it can be an easier decision, but we were starting from scratch if we were to do it again.

That meant all the harvesting and all the hormones we both had to take, etc. We really wanted children, so you bet we wanted to try it again. We didn't even mind spending the money again, so we tried a second time. This time we were successful in getting three fertilized eggs. We transferred two of them to Jennifer on the second try and unfortunately, neither of the eggs attached to the uterus. They absorbed, so we were not pregnant. We had one little egg hanging out there that was fertilized, which led to another discussion because we had said from the beginning we were going to do IVF two times only.

We were left with the option of having another egg available, but then that would be the third time, so then it was a question of whether we could be flexible on what we had decided. While we do set boundaries and put guidelines in, we shouldn't be so rigid as to not look at other alternatives. In our case, there's no way we could have personally and emotionally walked away from that last little egg without trying to see if it was "the one." So, we did.

It did not involve me taking hormones anymore, which was a good thing because I was starting to see side effects from them at that point. It did involve Jennifer taking hormones for a third time, so we decided to do IVF again. We transferred just that one egg and it also did not attach, so we didn't get pregnant that time either.

We chose a financial plan where we paid per treatment, not a flat fee. We spent tens of thousands of dollars. During times like this, when it's not successful, it's easy to feel like it's just money down the drain and money that could have been spent on something else or even in relation to time, it can be years that you could have been in the adoption process or doing something else. But, if you stay in that mindset, then it's not going to be productive to move forward especially if you want to have children.

So, have your pity party for a day; say all the things you need to say, cry out loud, be mad and scream at the top of your lungs about all the money you spent, all the time you put into it. Get all the emotions out and then get past it—get it away from you. Go from there so you can make good decisions as to whether you're going to choose another option or not.

Everyone Feels Loss Differently

After all of this, we did choose the adoption option, as do many people. But even while we were pursuing that, I started feeling different, not myself. I felt like I was going into a mild depression and my partner was continuing on her path, but didn't seem to feel the same way I felt or at least, didn't represent that we both felt the same way. I was talking to my friends and to Jennifer all the time about how I felt. I'm pretty outspoken on how I feel about just about everything, but nobody including myself (and I'm very self reflective) knew why I felt the way I felt or even the depths of how I felt.

Finding out why was critical in this stage, because unless I could determine why, I wasn't going to be able to pull myself out of it. The loss of potential pregnancy can have so many more affects on you then one would initially realize, because when you're reading this, you may be thinking to yourself, "You just lost a child, of course, you may become depressed." I realized that it was much deeper than that, but I didn't realize that until I went to counseling.

One of the situations I was having a problem with was that we were spending all this money on fertility. Well, I manage the finances in our household, and we were not doing well financially anymore. We were spending what we had to try to have children. At the office, I wasn't producing very well, because I had gotten to a point where I didn't care whether I showed up to work or not. I didn't care whether I had a client that day or not. What I also determined was that I felt out of control of my entire life, which came to a head when we lost our child. I had no control over the pregnancy. I had no control over the success of the fertilization of the eggs and whether they were going to attach inside the uterus, and I had no control over the loss.

Control was a big issue for me, and that was added to the financial stress. Through further counseling, I realized a loss of the expected life. I'm not talking about the loss of the child, but it was the expected child, the one I was going to have for years and years, and the joys and pain to be able to share with that child. I realized there was a real baby in there and that real baby was going to be mine to hold and to kiss, just like all the other people around me that I saw everywhere.

I didn't have that. I didn't have the stories I could then share with friends and family. But, that was all something I expected. What I didn't expect that I found through counseling was that I have not had a wonderful relationship with my own mother my whole life. She was my stepmother and became my mother when I was six years old. My father and birth mother were divorced when I was two and then my birth mother committed suicide when I was six, shortly after my father married my stepmother.

I wasn't divided between mothers. I had a step mother who was the only mother I knew, and we just didn't have a great relationship. A large part of that was because I was gay. When Jennifer and I got pregnant, as a couple, my mother started to become the mother that I had always wanted. She was very excited about having a grandchild. She went out and bought things for the baby.

I don't think I cognitively thought, "Yeah, this is the relationship I've been wanting." I sensed it and felt it, and I was hopeful that it would become the relationship that I wanted, but when we lost our child, while I didn't deliberately think, "Oh, now I've lost the relationship with my mother," deep down, that's what I was feeling. That's the loss I was mourning, more so than our child, on the long-term effects. The initial mourning was certainly for our child, but as it lingered and when I went through counseling, it was the loss of that relationship with my mother that I felt I wasn't going to have unless I had a child.

The Blessing of Support

I would never want a child solely for that purpose, but that was an added benefit I didn't even know about when we started creating our child. I certainly felt like a lead balloon when our child died, that I was losing the relationship with my mother. Through these experiences, there can be some wonderful awakenings if we are paying attention and if we get the awareness, either through ourselves or through the assistance of counseling that's available out there.

That's an experience that I had, which I found to be a positive experience through the loss of our child.

I believe a lot of men can identify with some of the feelings I was having after our loss when their wife has a miscarriage. Their pregnancy efforts are unsuccessful but they aren't the one carrying the child. After you lose your child, everyone asks the woman, the carrier of the baby, "How are you doing?"

Nobody asks the partner, the husband, that same thing—not in a way that is sincere and truly in the way that they ask the mother. It's "How is she coping with it? Is she doing okay? Really, how is she doing?" I started to get hurt that nobody was asking me how I was doing and I then became jealous because Jennifer was getting all the pampering, not in a superficial way, but true attention. Both of you go through the loss together, and you both have feelings, which is something I'm not even sure Jennifer realized was happening.

I was certainly quick to tell her about it, because I share everything, but I'm not so sure that men would share that with their wives. So, with this information, I'm hoping that people realize that men (and partners) are going through this process too and they need to be supported.

With everybody going through different emotions and processing their emotions differently, handling things in their own ways, sometimes the loss of a child or of an expectation can disrupt or destroy the relationship between the couple. What will maintain that relationship is mutual respect for each other's feelings, even if you don't understand exactly what they are going through. Throughout this time, Jennifer and I supported each other through thick and thin and when the time came for us to consider our second option, adoption, we were ready.

Poem About Adoption:
WE

A deed that's done
That which creates a little one
I'm too young you say
This was meant for a future day
But that day is here,
That day is now
To make a decision
But what and how?
To parent, to abort
Or to place your child in another's home?

Which of these choices
Will your family condone?
You will know what is right
Behind the tears you fight
When the future you see
Involves you, us and our baby as we.

After we had decided that we were not going to continue with fertility treatments, we immediately decided on adoption because we didn't know anything else. My best friend from Canada is adopted and Jennifer has a family member that we're very close with who was adopted. We felt we were a pretty good-looking couple and had a lot to offer given that we're both professionals. We live in a good city outside of a larger city, with a lot of diversity and culture; it's a great place to raise children. Our house was nice and it had enough bedrooms to accommodate everyone.

Once we made that decision and interviewed a lot of adoption agencies, we decided to choose one in our own geographical location. Another reason why we chose this agency was because so many agencies had their code words for not working with gay couples. We would be told that they only work with Christian couples; not that the two are mutually exclusive; however, that was how we were told that they would not work with us.

We go where we're wanted and welcomed, so we chose an adoptive parent focused adoption agency close to home that served all kinds of families and could help us. Our particular agency had well over 200 couples on the list to adopt a child. When it's open adoption, there is no true waiting list because the birth mother gets the applicable profiles and then chooses, but, of course, that doesn't mean you're not waiting.

Some people don't have a wait at all and other people wait years in that situation. We knew that we were going to be extremely proactive with the marketing of ourselves.

We did all of our homework as fast as we could so we could enter "the book" which means be put on the website. Our birth mother letter would then be put into the book for consideration. Once the birth mother letter was approved, we gave it to everyone (as we mentioned earlier in the Adoption section).

Meeting Sharon

During this process, we received a solid contact. This woman called us and was in the middle of deciding to move to Washington State. Her name was Sharon, and she said she didn't have any friends. She knew the birth father but he had abandoned her once he found out she was pregnant. She didn't have a job so she was going to move.

What was very helpful for us was that Sharon did not come through our agency, but we had our agency to bounce the situation off of. From the beginning, they started telling us this situation had a lot of red flags because she had stated that both of her parents died when she was young and that she had no friends, yet, she's about to move to another state. Also the fact that she knew the birth father, and stated that he had abandoned her. There were a lot of red flags as to whether this adoption was going to go forward.

To us, she seemed very sincere but in trouble. While there were a lot of red flags, it's also very typical of women who have unplanned pregnancies. Typically the male is not around. They are in lower socioeconomic status situations, which means that they may not have money for rent, and they're homeless, so they may be living in homeless shelters. Because of the choices they've made in their lives, they don't have a lot of family support and sometimes no friends.

We gave her the benefit of the doubt and were communicating with her. We started emailing back and forth. The emails turned into phone calls. We spent a few weeks talking about when we would meet and how we would meet and that's where another red flag presented itself. She kept delaying when we would meet in person.

Important: If a person is hesitant to meet you in person, even through an agency where it's facilitated and you're on a neutral and safe ground supported by agency counselors who know what they're doing, it may be a red flag that they're scamming you.

Ultimately she did decide to meet us. We flew out to Washington and we met. She was a beautiful professional woman who was in between jobs and she was living in a hotel in Washington. It was a nice hotel. We stayed there ourselves, so we knew what the nightly rates were. We moved the relationship forward, and she seemed to like us a lot, and we continued to call each other.

Watch the Scam Boards

Any time you are going through open adoption or doing it on your own, or if a birth mother contacts you and it's not through your agency specifically, you want to watch the scam boards. We entered some information to see if anyone had heard of Sharon. We also called an agency in the state where she had lived before she moved to Washington. Everything was telling us that Sharon was a scam. Nevertheless, we still maintained a relationship with her. It's important to have attorneys in the state where the adoption is going to occur, so we started interviewing some attorneys in Washington. Adoption is a small world, and there are few attorneys who specialize in that.

There were three attorneys focused on adoption law in the area of Washington where she was. I called two of them after Sharon and had agreed to match with us, which means you are planning on the same plan and that you will be adopting that child. We found out from two of the lawyers that she had already contacted them and was asking if they had prospective parent profiles for her to look through and decide if she wanted to meet with any of them. We felt very betrayed, like she had cheated on us and was continuing to cheat on us. We had to either walk away or raise the issue with her.

We did raise the issue, and she started crying, ultimately telling us that we didn't have a contract in place. We did not have a written contract in place and even if we did have a written contract, it is not legally binding as far as the ability to look for and match with other couples. It's a moral obligation and match, not a legal one.

We continued to talk with her for two to three weeks. It was a rollercoaster ride with some phone calls that were wonderful; she's courting us, we're courting her. There were other phone calls where she was just crying the whole time and telling us she doesn't know what to do. We were trying to be supportive of her while knowing she was still talking with other couples.

We started thinking, "Should we continue to hang on or stop this relationship? If the other couples find out that she's talking to us, maybe they'll walk away first, and she'll be left with no one but us and by default, we'll win."

We did have the communication with the lawyers of those clients. She had met with some of them and one lawyer said that he was going to tell his client not to work with this birth mother. The other lawyer decided to let the best couple win. We knew there was a lawyer out there who was going to continue showing prospective couples, even knowing that we were out there and that Sharon had matched with us.

What We Learned
• • • • • • • • • • • • • • • • • • •

Ultimately, we found out that she had been kicked out of the hotel. We decided the situation was too turbulent for us and we walked away. That was an adoption situation that did not go to full-term.

Even though we saw all the signs from the beginning, with our agency telling us this situation is not one they recommend, we did it anyway. Many couples will continue to pursue the hope of that child. Besides the situation not working out, once you match with a birth mother, you are taken out of the adoption book. You cannot be presented to any other birth mother situations. They could be perfect and true non-scammers, a situation where someone is truly committed to the process, but you just aren't eligible.

We were taken out of the book for a while and that's okay because we had to go through this process. Many couples do. I would suggest if you want your child in 12 months or less, and you're using an adoption agency, listen to the advisors that you have around you. If they tell you it has a very high risk for scam opportunities, listen to them and look for the next opportunity.

The Biggest Take-Away We Got

The worst thing you can do is blame yourself as to why it did not work out or start asking if it was something you said or did. It's not productive or helpful. It's not you, but the situation, so move on. Get back on the horse and wait for more calls. Continue to do your networking and marketing.

Time to Bring in the Adoption Facilitator

After that situation had fallen through, we decided that our agency and our marketing efforts weren't going quick enough for us, so we hired an adoption facilitator. We brought this up earlier where we had a recommendation from a friend of mine who had used her. My friend was the first client this adoption facilitator had. The facilitator had a child in my friend's hands within two days of when she hired her.

I thought that was awesome. Of course, this is not typical results, but someone I knew personally had extremely good results with a facilitator. When I contacted and interviewed her, she told me that she maintained no more than 10 prospective parents as clients at any given time. She also explained how she reached out to the adoption agencies that focus on birthmothers as well as social workers, doctors, and OBGYN's.

Why We Felt She Was Reputable

At any given time, you could go to her website and see all available situations that needed parents to be matched with birth mothers. You could also see the price it would cost, and see which ones had been matched already.

We went to the website and saw the available situations. We thought it looked good. As far as fees, she was a bit higher because there may be other agencies involved. In researching for this Chapter, I recently went to her website again and she had five available situations and two matched situations. The range of fees was between $29,000 and $45,000. While high, we know for a fact that the birthmother is a person who is either pregnant or has already had the child and is committed to the adoption situation.

When I say committed, you don't know until the papers are signed by the judge that there is a true commitment, but these are people who have been heavily screened by agencies, so they will let you know if there are red flags or not. Within the first month of hiring the adoption facilitator, we had been presented two situations that met our profile. We were not chosen by either of those and then were presented to a third situation. It was, in our mind, the perfect match.

Texas and the Aries Baby

The situation was the birthmother was pregnant with a baby girl, which is what we had been pregnant with. This child was full Caucasian.

She was to be born in Texas, which is where I am from. If you know anything about Texans, we're very proud of our state and heritage.

Because the child would be born there, the adoption laws of the state where the child is born rule. In Texas, there is a 48-hour waiting period before the birthmother can sign relinquishments. After 48 hours the birthmother cannot change her mind. There is no re-claim period.

Why it Sounded Like a Match

The shorter the re-claim period the better for the couple that wants to adopt because it's much less stressful. The child was going to be born in April, which is the month that I was born in. I like Aries babies. I am biased there. On paper, it couldn't have been better. Oh, and the birthmother specifically wanted a lesbian couple because her mother was lesbian, as well. Her mother was very supportive of the adoption plan.

What Happened

We were notified two weeks before the due date that this birthmother was looking to place her child for adoption. She had been working with an agency for about three months, so it wasn't a decision she made overnight. She had decided to finalize what couple she wanted. Once we were notified, we sent our profile book. She said she wanted to meet us so we flew to Texas. I can tell you, a flight from Georgia to Texas when you book it today to fly tomorrow is not inexpensive, especially with two of you. Not to mention, we were flying back the same day we flew in.

We flew down, had dinner with the birthmother, the birthmother's mother, and the agency social worker. We matched, she chose us, and it was very good. We took pictures because it was important to us to memorialize the whole situation for our child's sake. The other wonderful thing for us was that it was a short courtship. We didn't have to spend months wondering if she really liked us, if we were saying the right things, how often we should call, etc. With this one, it was two weeks until the due date.

The Day of the Birth

When she went into labor, the agency called us, and we went to the hospital. We stayed all night for the birth, which happened some time in the early morning. Because of the 48-hour period, the birthmother stayed in the hospital the full two days after the birth, which I find interesting now given that women who have healthy babies can go home the same day. In fact, the hospitals generally push you out the same day.

Our birthmother stayed in the hospital the full two days. The baby stayed in the hospital the full two days and during that time we spent a lot of time getting to know the birthmother and her mother. We spent both days holding the baby girl, feeding her, changing her and we felt like we were in tune with the birthmother and the experience she was going through.

In that 48 hours, she decided to parent and changed her mind on the adoption. We were waiting at our hotel room. On the day we were going to take the child home with us, we were to meet at 10:00 a.m. at the hospital. At 9:00 a.m., we had packed everything, and were getting ready to leave for the hospital when we got a phone call.

The Phone Call

It was the social worker from the agency. She told us not to come to the hospital because the birthmother had changed her mind. We were on the phone with the social worker who didn't work for us. We wanted to ask questions. "How sure are you? Is there anything you can do to convince her not to change her mind?"

It was not her job to convince a birthmother to do one thing or the other. It was to be there to support the birthmother in whatever her decision was. The social worker wasn't providing any support to us on the phone. We were just told the birthmother had changed her mind and that we would receive a call back to let us know where to go from there. She did call us back an hour later, which was the 48th hour, and advised us that the birthmother had already left the hospital with the child.

The Aftermath

As a couple that felt that we bonded with that child for two days, we didn't have a chance to say goodbye. At the very least, we wanted to explain that we cared a lot for the child, and tell the child that we cared for her and that we wished her very well in her life. Therefore, that child, who has some sense of awareness that we were in her life for two days, would have some closure and certainly for personal reasons, we wanted our own closure. It would also have been good to have closure with the birth mother, as well.

We got the sense and feeling that the attitude was, "Thanks for coming. Go home now. You're not needed here anymore."

When you adopt a child in another state, you have to stay in that state for a period of time, and it can be up to two weeks. Our plane ticket back was not for a while, so we decided to stay. We were hanging out waiting.

When something like this happens, you may have a little too much time on your hands, and may not be spending it in the most productive way. You may see a side of yourself that you never knew existed.

We wanted to take all the clothes and the baby items that we purchased and give them to the birthmother as a gift before we decided to return them. That is what we probably would have done if we were able to go to the hospital that morning to say goodbye. We would have given her those things. We believe they were intended to be for this child. They would have been a present from us. I was feeling benevolent towards her.

But, we didn't have that chance to say goodbye. My benevolent feelings turned around, and then I wanted to throw everything at her. I wanted to go to her house and leave them all over her yard and tell her that she didn't deserve them and that she certainly couldn't provide for the child the way we could.

Obviously, those are not healthy or productive actions. They may be healthy and cathartic to get out of me so I can move forward through my anger, but they weren't good. Jennifer and I were going through the five stages of loss and anger was one of them. You just don't know the depth of what your mind processes and what you can go through when you're so angry.

Then I wanted to write her a letter and beg her to come to her senses. She was under the age of 18. I wanted her to come to her senses and realize that she's just a child. She couldn't raise this child like we could.

A Time for Questions
••••••••••••••••••••••

I can't speak for Jennifer, but I personally doubted all belief I had in God and what that meant to me, and I wondered why this could all be happening. Were we not supposed to have children at all? Was it something I did in my childhood? Had I not repented for something I had done? What could be out there that's preventing me from having a child, preventing Jennifer and me, as a couple, from having a child?

We still had to board a plane and carry the empty car seat that we had taken from Georgia to Texas to bring our baby home. You cannot leave the hospital without a car seat.

You start wondering if you said the wrong things; were you too eager to adopt this child? You project what you're friends and family at home are going to say because they have observed the entire process if you've allowed them into your life enough to observe the joys as well as the sorrows.

You start thinking that it will never work out. You think that maybe you should give up and stop putting yourself through this. *"What has changed? I knew this would never work."* Your support system probably won't say things like that, but you're thinking that they're thinking those things. I do have a family member who did say they never had a good feeling about that situation, which did not shock me because she shared that along the way, as well.

Then you have friends who have successfully adopted a child or children. If you've heard it once, you've head it a million times, "You know when it's right. You can feel it when it's right." Everyone who has adopted a child will say that.

Well, it's easy to say that on the backend when you have the child, but when you're going through it, honestly, you don't know anything until the judge signs the paper. You don't know shit. If there were ever a situation that could have been more right, it was the one in Texas. It hit every element. We were there and on the same vibration, and it didn't work.

Just be aware that people will say this to you. This is a time when you may want to have a nice canned response that you can say. "When it's right, it will happen." If we want it to be right, it's going to be right in our minds and in our feelings. There is so much at play that until the judge signs the order; you will not know it's right. You can hope that it's going to turn out the way you would like it to.

To this day, even though I now have two wonderful children, I still cry thinking about that adoption process. Jennifer has shared that she feels that after two days bonding with that child, talking with that child, caring for and loving the child that she felt that was more difficult than when we lost our child after the amniocentesis. She felt the child was real and born, whereas our child was only an expectation of a child.

Self-Reflection and Transparent Beliefs

I felt myself slipping back into the mild depression that I had after we lost our first child. I knew that I didn't want to go there again. I wanted to do whatever I could to maintain a positive, healthy mind, so we did something about it.

There is a certain philosophy that teaches you through certain tools how to find any hidden beliefs that you may have that you don't know about. They're called transparent beliefs. The reason you don't know you have them is because you've piled so many other beliefs on top of them through experiences you've gone through.

I wanted to find out if I had any beliefs about having children that was preventing me from doing so. Jennifer and I went through this process together. Well actually we went through the same process, but it is an individual reflection. We each went through the process on our own to see if we had any transparent beliefs.

Jennifer realized through her process that she had a belief that having children is hard and that it's not an easy process. As long as she had that belief she would inadvertently or subconsciously create a situation that was making it difficult to be successful having a child.

The Big Ah-Ha!

I had a transparent belief that I discovered only through going through this technique and that was that: *I believe that mommies should keep their babies.*

When you find a transparent belief, it's not a thinking exercise; it's a feeling exercise. You know it's the true belief you have because you have either an emotional or physical reaction once that belief surfaces. Even before I could get it out of my mouth I started sobbing uncontrollably.

It was so profound for me. As soon as I felt that, I knew exactly why I felt that way.

If I had a belief that mommies should keep their babies, there could have been 100 adoption situations that presented themselves to us and unconsciously (or through my energy) I would have prevented those adoptions from being successful.

How did I get that belief and why would I feel that way if I were so supportive of adoption? The only explanation I had that I feel is 100% true was that my mother and father got divorced when I was two years old, and my father got custody of us. It didn't appear to me, throughout my life that my mother had fought hard enough to keep us. So, subconsciously, if I saw a baby that was going to either be given away or kept with its mother, I would choose the latter as the ideal scenario.

Another Light Bulb

Jennifer and I decided we were not going to pursue adoption any further. I didn't want to go through any more depression if I could avoid that. It was like a light bulb went off, and I remembered that a colleague of mine and I had lunch one day. I was sharing with him our efforts to have a child and he shared with me that he and his wife had gone through the exact same infertility issues.

They had a couple of miscarriages. They had gone through the adoption process, held a baby in their arms that was ripped away. Then they chose surrogacy. They had a successful situation, which resulted in a child through surrogacy. At the time of our lunch conversation, they were pregnant with twins through a surrogate. Even though we had that lunch and discussion earlier in the process, it didn't click for me because I wasn't that familiar with surrogacy. There are no billboards out there describing it.

After the second failed adoption and after we had gone through the self-reflection exercise, I was sitting in my office focusing on babies. The light bulb went on, and I knew I needed to get back in touch with my colleague. I needed to ask him more about his experience with surrogacy.

What do you think about Surrogacy?

I did and he told me everything there was that he had gone through. I went home. Jennifer and I walk our dog every night and I asked her what she thought about surrogacy. She told me she would have to think about it, and I told her she had to think fast because I'd already contacted six women who were interested or available to help us with surrogacy and they were waiting for our response. That is how we were led to the next process.

Getting to Baby Surrogacy Story: Victory!

I called my colleague who had used a surrogate, and we talked on the phone for quite a while. I was at my office and he was at his. He told me again about how a surrogate had pretty much landed in his lap through his professional line of work.

He explained how the process went, and shared about the pregnancy and how joyful they were to have a child.

"As a matter of fact, after some time had gone by after the birth of our first child, the surrogate came back to us asking if we wanted to have more children. She told us that she would like to help us again if we were interested," he told me with enthusiasm in his voice.

So, at the time when he and I were talking, he was pregnant through the surrogate with twins. He told me about www.surromomsonline.com. While he didn't personally use them, one of his colleagues was going through surrogacy and had found a surrogate there.

"Well, this has been incredibly helpful and inspiring. Thank you!" I felt like I couldn't get off the phone quick enough; while I was very interested in his story, once I knew the direction I needed to go, I just wanted to go on the website and start looking around.

Research and Responses

I spent the next five hours researching and looking at the ads from the potential surrogates. I emailed six women via the website and told them a bit about our situation because again, I was already in tune with what the code language was, so I tried to select women that looked like they would be a good fit for our situation.

While I stayed away from those looking for Christian couples, I did contact some that said they would help gay men. I thought if they were flexible enough to be able to work with gay men, maybe they would consider us, as a lesbian couple.

Of the six that I reached out to, we received three responses. Two of them were out of state and one was in state. One of them was a lesbian couple that wanted to be a surrogate for a gay couple; she had never even considered doing it for a lesbian couple. We did not choose them for a few reasons. They were out of state and the one who was going to be the surrogate wanted to be a traditional surrogate, which meant she wanted to use her own egg.

The other potential surrogate who was out of state lived in a state that bordered Georgia—North Carolina. She was married, had her own children, and she had already been a surrogate. She was looking for the right fit, but her time schedule wasn't what our time schedule was, in that she wanted to take it very slowly; she wanted to build up a relationship first and then ease into it.

While building up the relationship was something that was important to us, we also were on a time schedule, not only because we wanted to have children before we were 40, but also because we had been through so many processes. At this point, we just wanted to get someone who was ready to begin and were as eager as we were.

Brittany
• • • • • • • • •

That someone was our third person that we contacted; her name was Brittany. She lived in Georgia. We emailed back and forth. There was also a picture of her on www.surromomsonline.com. While it seems silly, we're all attracted to people for various reasons, even in non-sexual ways. We are drawn to people we become friends with; there's something that attracts us to that person and them to us. That was the case for us with Brittany; the first thing we noticed in her picture was that she had the most beautiful blue eyes.

Brittany posted her ad saying that she was looking for intended parents. I can only imagine how scary, yet how exciting that must be. Just like intended parents who are putting an ad out there, it's very exciting because you're embarking on a whole new world, but too, it's scary because you don't know if somebody is going to respond, you don't know who is going to respond or what will go on from there.

It was the day after she had posted her ad when I responded to it. She said something that really tugged at my heart strings. She mentioned that nobody had contacted her first day of posting her ad. It was obvious that she was feeling vulnerable.

She said in her post, "Why hasn't anyone contacted me?" When I read that, I thought, "She feels the way I have always felt through the adoption process." "Why aren't they contacting us? What is it about me?" It was just so endearing in the sweetest way. We were immediately drawn to her and were just hoping that our meeting would go well, and it did.

Even though we weren't planning on using her eggs, we reconsidered. She was tall. We knew we wanted to have twins if at all possible, so her size was important to us as far as being able to carry twins successfully. I'm 5'3" and barely weigh 100 lbs. I would not want to birth twins. We wanted someone who felt that they could.

She responded to our email, and we started talking on the phone. We arranged a meeting and met within two weeks of our initial conversation. That was in May of 2009. She had two children and was a single mom. We wanted to make it most accommodating for her, so we drove to where she lived and met at a restaurant for lunch on neutral ground and made sure it was a very non-threatening meeting. These are things that should be taken into consideration when meeting a stranger, for the security and safety of the potential surrogate as well as for the intended parents.

The Match

We knew immediately that we just loved her. She seemed to really take to us, as well. She was shy, certainly not as outspoken as I am, and she was very sweet and wholesome. After having gone through some potential adoption scams and as lawyers, we were just skeptical by nature, but it just felt right. We matched.

She said she wanted to work with us, and we wanted to work with her. We had already drafted a preliminary contract, but it wasn't exactly what we would have signed. It just had some terms spelled out. Right there at the table, we outlined on a piece of paper what we were going to agree to or at least the backbone of what we were going to agree to. The three of us signed that piece of paper, so it felt like a contract where we were formally matched with each other.

Moving Closer
• • • • • • • • • • • • •

Brittany wanted to move out of her town, and we wanted someone closer to us, so we agreed to move her up close to where we were.

She moved up to Atlanta within two weeks of our first meeting. We have some friends who invest in real estate, and they had a vacant home that needed a tenant so we moved Brittany and her children into that home for a month. During that month, we purchased a foreclosed home, and we fixed it up quickly so it was livable and nice; she moved in the next month into a house that we purchased and owned.

One reason why we liked that situation is that we could control the costs of what the living arrangement would be. Given that she had just moved to a new city, she wouldn't have the availability to find a job easily, especially in this economy.

We didn't particularly want her to work outside the home because we didn't want her to worry about daycare, taking care of her children and all of those decisions. Making money to provide for her would cause potential stress on her body, which could then lead to stress for the pregnancy and maybe even prevent pregnancy. We just wanted things to be as easy, smooth and as stress-free as possible and to be able to control expenses.

Since we were already doing real estate investing, this added to our portfolio. We were basically killing two birds with one stone, as I like to say. We wanted a close relationship. She was living in a house we owned, living in the same city as we were in and also, since I own my own business, I was able to employ her on a part-time basis where she could work from home and earn some of her own money.

Setting Parameters
• • • • • • • • • • • • • • • • • • •

We developed a close relationship. Doing that can also come with risks, especially when you're that tied to each other. The surrogate can become very dependent on the intended parents, especially if the intended parents are taking care of everything.

For example, we were the landlords. If something went wrong in the house, we were called; we had to go mow the yard, change the air filter, and change the little plumbing kit in the back of the toilet. All of those things happened while she was living there. Those are issues that people have to be careful of—the surrogate becoming too dependent on the intended parents.

It can certainly go the other way. Like I said, I had employed her part-time in my law firm. It could have been a situation where I didn't want her to stop working after the pregnancy was over. Issues like that can come up so those are the kinds of things when you're looking at a relationship with a surrogate, you have to decide how close is close enough and how close is too close? You have to set parameters on that relationship.

Because surrogacy is fertility under another name, we did go through the same IVF fertility process that Jennifer and I used from the very beginning with our own process. With Brittany, she was the one taking the medication; she was the patient of the clinic, so Jennifer and I were in a supportive role through the fertility process.

We went to every single doctor's appointment as if Brittany were our own partner. There were times when Brittany had a doctor's appointment and Jennifer or I would be like, "I don't want to go to this one. Can you go to this one, and I'll go to the next one?"

We knew that if it were one of us that were pregnant, the other would be there no matter what. So, we treated Brittany exactly the same way unless we had another conflict and just could not change plans.

The Process
• • • • • • • • • • •

As mentioned, she moved to Atlanta two weeks after we met. Within the next 30 days, we did all of the medical and psychological testing that's required, and we synched her menstrual cycle for a particular date of transfer. Because we were purchasing frozen eggs, we didn't have to synch her menstrual cycle up with another female; it was just a matter of counting the days as to when she was going to have a menstrual cycle so they could thaw the eggs and fertilize the egg with the sperm at the right time.

We purchased nice, healthy young eggs and nice, healthy, young clean sperm and several fertilized. We chose to transfer two embryos into Brittany.

A sign of a good and ethical fertility clinic is a doctor that will not transfer more than two embryos at a time. Our doctor was one of those. He knew from the beginning that we wanted twins, so we transferred two embryos. Within 10 days, I believe is when we can get our blood test for the pregnancy, and we had a very positive pregnancy test.

We all went to the doctor for the blood test. When the pregnancy test results are ready, they call you on the phone to tell you. These decisions are very interesting because the intended parents are the ones who are "getting pregnant." The surrogate is the patient, so the clinic would normally call the patient with the results.

Our surrogate was so respectful of our situation that she told them to call us. Jennifer and I scheduled a time when we could both be available via phone, so the clinic called us and then we called Brittany and told her. It was a very unique and interesting situation.

Prior to the day that we did the transfer, Brittany had done some research on the Internet and found the coolest t-shirts that showed the stick from a home pregnancy test on the front of it with the bars indicating positive pregnancy results. On the t-shirt, it said "Positive

Thoughts." Because of our relationship and because we were able to go to all the doctor appointments together, it allowed us to really bond. We purchased the shirts for all three of us to wear on the day of transfer.

When we walked in, the whole doctor's office saw it, and they were enlightened, in a good mood, and cheery; that's the kind of mood you want on a day like that. You want confidence and calmness. That was a fun day for us.

After the positive pregnancy test, Brittany disclosed that she knew all along because she had been peeing on a stick since day three.

Everything Doesn't Always Go As Planned

The pregnancy became very difficult. Just because you hire a surrogate, it doesn't mean you're out of the water, even if the surrogate has had very easy pregnancies in the past.

With our situation, the pregnancy was going great at first; when we went back to our doctor for blood tests, her levels to indicate pregnancy just kept doubling, so we had an indication even before we could have an ultrasound that the likelihood was multiples; hopefully, just twins and no more than twins for our situation and for our own desires.

When we went in for the first ultrasound, the three of us went together. That was with the OBGYN that we had chosen, the same OBGYN that Jennifer and I had used who knew that we had gone through the adoption process, did the amniocentesis with us and knew that we had lost our child, so this was a great event. For us to be at our OBGYN who had seen us through everything was really special. She was showing us the two little blips on the screen that represented the heartbeats. Everything was going great.

We got past the 12-week critical stage, then past the 17 weeks where Jennifer and I had our amniocentesis and lost our child in the previous try. With this pregnancy, we did not choose to do an amniocentesis because we had a young surrogate, young eggs and young sperm.

Then, at 20 weeks Brittany's cervix started to turn outward. The doctor put her on bed rest at home. We aren't talking light bed rest; it was total bed rest. She has two children at home so that's not easy when the children are both under the age of three years old; there's a lot of picking up, following after and things that parents have to do.

The Benefits of Us Planning Ahead

In our contract, which is why contracts are so important, we had already outlined what to do if Brittany went on bed rest or was in the hospital. In our contract, we had agreed to pay for childcare. We hired a home healthcare company that provides nurses aides for the children. I chose a company that I had used for my elderly clients, which made it convenient because it was last minute.

Ultimately, there were issues with that so Brittany's sister needed to be moved up to live in the home, which was a great support system for Brittany. When I talk about the need for support systems, it's not just about us as the intended parents, but the surrogate needs support as well.

We also had to hire a housekeeper because when someone is on bed rest, they can't maintain their house the same way they did when they were healthy.

She was on bed rest for three weeks doing what the doctor said. We went into another doctor's appointment at week 23, which is just over four months of pregnancy. At that appointment, the ultrasound showed that the embryonic fluid sac that surrounds the babies, the one closest to the cervix was protruding through the cervix, into the vagina.

The sac is made up of thin membranes and very fragile. Brittany was admitted into the hospital directly from the doctor's appointment. Emergency arrangements for her children had to be made. At this point, her sister had not yet moved up, and we still had the home healthcare givers.

Jennifer and I were at the doctor's appointment with Brittany; I stayed with her and made sure the admission to the hospital went well. Jennifer was making accommodations for the children and trying to get an emergency caregiver there overnight, because we hadn't had to make any overnight arrangements to this point, so all of that had to be taken care of.

Cervical Cerclage

We got Brittany admitted into the hospital. The plan was that she would essentially lie on her head for three days in a hospital bed that is tilted head down at a particular angle. The idea was that gravity would pull the sac back into the uterus where it's supposed to be. When that happened, they would do a surgical procedure called Cervical Cerclage to sew up the cervix so that nothing could protrude through it.

I spent the first night on the couch in Brittany's hospital room, as Brittany had to lie in the bed. She had a serious nosebleed. Hanging head down like she was can cause you to get lightheaded, a huge headache and sometimes nose bleeds. Brittany had all those issues.

The next day, she started having extreme pain. They believed it was the issue with the sac, but she ended up having a gallstone that she had to pass. What better place to do this then at the hospital?

But it could have interfered with the whole idea of the sac going where it was supposed to go. At the end of the three days, the sac was not moving. She had another ultrasound, and it was in the same place it was before. This pregnancy had become termed extremely high risk for pre-term labor and loss of the children, because at 23 weeks children cannot live outside the body, generally speaking.

The night before the procedure for the cerclage, which is a surgical procedure, the hospital told us that the neonatal specialists were going to come talk to us but didn't really explain why or what the discussion was going to be about.

So, this doctor comes, and we're all in the room together. Everyone kept calling Brittany "mom," and she kept saying, "I'm not the mother, they're the mothers; talk to them. They'll be making these decisions." Even though it was her body, she respected that it was our decision with regard to what to do about the procedures. She was actually quite offended throughout the whole process when someone did make a mistake and refer to her as the mom.

This is not like adoption. She never intended to be the mother. It wasn't her egg, so it's a different mindset for a surrogate. We were very blessed that she had that opinion.

Decision Time

The doctor is talking to us. It becomes very clear after an hour of him talking to us and us just sitting there listening, that what he has said without saying it is these babies are potentially going to die tomorrow if the procedure isn't successful. He stopped talking at one moment and just sat there.

He didn't ask us a question or anything; he just sat there. I looked at Jennifer, and she looked at me. Then I looked at the doctor and said, "Are you saying that, right now, we need to decide if this procedure is not successful if we want life support for our children or not?" He looked at us and said, "Yes, that's what I need to know."

We told him we did want the life support if necessary and then we'd make a decision as to whether we wanted to continue it or not. An hour discussion of what all the risks are is not enough time for us to fully develop a plan for the rest of our lives or theirs. That was an interesting situation and discussion but one that was very necessary.

Not Again!

It was the first time that we had an indication that we may lose these children. Then a perinatologist who had been doing all of our high risk ultrasounds, which at this point we started having weekly, came in and said, "We're going to do this." At this point, we started feeling like we were losing control of the situation and the decision-making process.

The doctor said they were going to go in and look. If it was still coming through, they were going to push it back up and try to do the surgery. I asked, "Don't we have any input on these decisions? Can't you come out and consult with us? Aren't we the ones who get to make that decision?"

"Brittany is going to be unconscious during this procedure so it's not like you can ask her on the table. Can't you come back and ask us before you push it up there or do whatever you need to do?" The doctor told us that it was their decision because when they're in there they wouldn't have time to come and talk to us.

The Fun Doctor

They wheeled Brittany down the next morning and the doctor came in. At this point, we had sort of a fun relationship with the doctor. He fortunately, was one of the kinds of doctors who was very relaxed, very calm and joking in good and tactful ways while being very professional.

I always had questions. I don't think doctors expect that. I think that most people just accept information that they're given; they don't know what to ask, don't know that they can ask and sometimes they feel that they're questioning the doctor's authority if they ask questions. I don't. I think I have the right to understand everything before letting something proceed even if I don't have the decision to say yes or no to proceed, I at least have the ability to know what's going on.

After all we had been through, I felt strongly about this. Every single process brought its own new, unique challenge that we had never heard of before. We were researching every aspect about a cerclage for three days. I actually could competently ask him, "Which procedure are you going to use?" because there are multiple types of ways to do this surgery.

On the day of the procedure, he came in and asked if we had any questions. I said, "No, I don't." He looked at me in surprise, and I said, "Well, actually, I do. What did you have for breakfast this morning?" He told me. The surgery was scheduled for 1:00 p.m. so, I said, "What are you going to have for lunch?" He told me what he was going to have for lunch. I also asked, "Did you have a fight with your wife or anyone else this morning?"

I didn't care about his credentials anymore because I knew he was the best. I wanted to know, how he was doing that day. "Is your mood going to affect this surgery at all? Is your appetite, are you going to be hungry and wishing you had eaten while you were down there doing what you need to do?"

Not only was it a serious question, but I think it also lightened the mood, at least for him, if not for us. Those things are very important. You don't want somebody building your car on a Friday afternoon; there are actually reports out there about that.

I didn't want my doctor having surgery on an empty stomach or after having a fight with his wife. All of that was good and after lunch he came to tell us what he ate and that it was nutritious.

The Waiting Game

We had to go to the same waiting room as everybody else who is waiting for different kinds of medical procedures—some are life threatening and some are not. You're waiting and waiting, and you just don't know how long it will take. Specifically, they tell you what an average may take if there are no complications so then, of course, when you reach that average, and they're not still out there, you can only assume that there are complications.

Jennifer and I are in the waiting room; it was very reminiscent of the time when we lost our own child in that, at that moment, during the waiting period, there was nothing Jennifer and I could say to each other; we had no amount of control over the situation at this point.

Moment of Truth

In fact, there was a time that I literally sat in my seat and said to myself, "God it's all you now; there's nothing I can do; there are no more prayers I have or that I could even say. I'm giving it up. If I'm supposed to have children, I am. If I'm not, I'm not, because this is our last attempt. I surrender to You." There was no bargaining or pleading, only surrender.

Shortly thereafter, the doctor came walking out into the waiting room. He sat down right next to us instead of taking us to the private waiting room where he could talk privately to us. He explained that the surgery was successful. We just started crying for joy and release of tension.

He thought he was off the hook, but he wasn't because I wanted to know everything that happened during the surgery. I don't know why I needed to know, but I did. So he sat there and explained it all. He told us that they pushed the sac back up with a little gauze and then they sewed up the cervix.

We found out later when we were making a documentary about our situation that our OBGYN stated that 99% of the time in this particular procedure, the way they had to do it, the sac breaks and the pregnancy is lost. So, we are extremely blessed that ours was successful.

Back to Brittany

After the cerclage was put in, Brittany had to stay in the hospital for five weeks on complete bed rest. Her sister moved in and became a full-time caregiver to Brittany's children. Brittany's sister didn't have any of her own children. In fact, her sister was several years younger than Brittany, so she really took on a role that none of us expected. Not only did we have a great support system, but Brittany had such great support, as well. It's beneficial to the situation for the surrogate to have that kind of support.

Jennifer and I were visiting Brittany at the hospital just about every day because we were her only family and her only support system that could visit. That was also an interesting situation because the OBGYN was calling us to ask for information as to whether he should release her to go home. Should she stay, based on the home environment, based on whether she could in fact, stay on bed rest at home versus taking care of her children.

All of those issues were factors on how long she had to stay in the hospital, but after she had been there for five weeks, we had reached the 28th week of pregnancy. At 28 weeks, babies can live outside the body. They are viable, so you've met another hurdle as to viability and lowering the risk of losing the pregnancy and the children.

Her Body, Our Children

Brittany was discharged to go home, but she was still on bed rest. This is where it became very difficult for us as far as the dimension of, this is her body, she gets to choose what she does with it, and these are our children. We almost lost them; we didn't want anything to risk this pregnancy from this point forward.

Even if they're born at 28 weeks, there is a much higher risk of physical and mental disabilities since their organs are not developed yet. We have very different lifestyles from each other, so some internal conflicts came into play.

As intended parents, you just have to trust that it's all going to be okay, so keep your mouth shut, keep your eyes on the babies and continue to be supportive of what the surrogate is going through.

Baby Showers

Once people knew the babies were okay, some of them wanted to throw baby showers for us. Through the adoption process we learned that you don't have a shower until that baby is home with you and the judge's order is signed. With the surrogacy, we felt more comfortable with regard to having a baby shower before the babies were born, but we certainly wanted to wait until as many of the medical issues as possible were behind us.

We had two different baby showers. Interestingly, the very first one we had on a Sunday afternoon. We invited Brittany to come.

That's a big question—do you invite your surrogate to the baby shower? Is that an encroachment on you and your excitement because it's not really about her? Or, do you not invite her? Will she feel left out?

We made the decision to invite Brittany because we felt that this was a process for the three of us. While these are not her children, she certainly can also be joyous and celebrate the occasion with us. She did come to our baby shower, but at the very first one, we were concerned because she seemed to be set off by herself. People tried to talk with her, and she was social—not near as social as I am, but she just seemed to be uncomfortable, and we were concerned. What happened the following day explained why.

We had a doctor's appointment the very next day, and she was admitted to the hospital. We had a perinatal appointment on Tuesday and they decided to induce labor because her blood pressure was so high that she was a serious risk for stroke. She was bloated, which is why she was uncomfortable at the baby shower. It didn't have anything to do with her attending the shower and it not being her occasion. Think about those issues, because those issues come up when there are three of you instead of two.

We are very glad that we invited her to the shower. We had two showers because we had two very different groups of friends. At the second shower, the babies were already born, but were in the NICU at the hospital. Our friends asked us if we wanted a second shower, and we thought this was the best time to have it because the babies are at the hospital, Brittany had been discharged, and we had some time on our hands.

At the second baby shower, Brittany felt much more comfortable because she wasn't about to explode with our two children. We opened all of the gifts for the children. Jennifer and I had decided that this was a true process for the three of us to celebrate so we waited until the very last moment of the gift opening, and we presented a gift to Brittany.

Just like wanting to create a special moment for her leaving the hospital with the limousine, we also wanted to create a special moment for her in front of our friends. We wanted her to know that what she had done for us was not just recognized by us, but that our friends appreciated it, as well.

So, we gave her a necklace that had one pink and one blue sapphire to represent our babies (one female and one male) that she carried for us. That was our symbol of thank you and remembrance of the two children that she carried for us, especially through such a difficult pregnancy.

The Big Day: Countdown to Baby

Getting back to the birth, we went to a normal weekly doctor's appointment, and the doctor said, "I'm going to admit you today and we're going to induce these children." Our OBGYN was just wonderful. He and his wife had twins around 20+ years before.

From the day we met Brittany until the day she was being induced, Brittany's intent, her only desire was to have a vaginal birth. Not a natural birth, which means without medication, but she wanted a vaginal birth if, at all possible.

This was only one of two doctors in the entire metro Atlanta area that we knew of that would honor her desire and not at the very last minute make up an excuse as to why they would have to do a C-section. I knew the doctor personally as well, not just professionally, so that made it much nicer.

When we had these complications, he did not stress out outwardly. He did not tell us, "Oh my God, she's about to have a stroke. We need to get her in there." The entire time he continued to let us know that most likely she would be able to have a vaginal birth because baby A, the first one to come out, was head down the entire pregnancy.

Three days before the doctor's appointment, Brittany had felt Baby B shift and was also head down. So, unless anything changed or because of the high risk part of the pregnancy, meaning that if they had to go to a C-section for any reason, then she was going to have her vaginal birth.

When we were in the labor room, they did all the regular procedures to induce. They put her on medication to start the labor. Then she wanted medication to not feel the labor pains. They wound up giving her too much, and she felt like she was paralyzed from the eyeballs down. The only thing she could move was her eyeballs. She was in a massive amount of pain. Looking back now, it was a bit comical but in that room, it seemed very serious, and there was just nothing we could do for her.

She blogged about her entire pregnancy experience as she was going through it. I remembered she blogged that when her gall bladder hurt, we just stood there in the room and stared at her like she was a freak or something. But, in a situation like that, you rely on what the doctors can do, and there's nothing else, you can do. So at this moment, having read that blog, I just kept thinking that she is going to feel like we're just standing here staring at her.

Then we had brought all of the cameras in because we had been recording the entire relationship and pregnancy; we certainly wanted to get the birth because we were making a documentary. Brittany was in pain, couldn't move, and we had this video camera staring at her. That was how we went into labor. The doctor came in and at some point decided they were going to break the sac and not wait for it to break on its own. At that point, we didn't know the severity of her blood pressure, but we did know that it was high.

We saw the contractions on the monitors, so we saw that they were getting close. A nurse came in and broke the water while the doctor kept popping in. At one point he mentioned he was going to take a nap because he felt it would take a couple more hours before she was ready. He seemed to be very laid back.

Ready for Their Close-Ups: Christopher and Katherine

Then when the event came, I had the video camera in one hand and Jennifer was standing by with the regular camera. The doctor told us we were involved and that we needed to hold Brittany's legs back. He needed us to pull them back so he could do his thing and she could relax and push the way she's supposed to without having to worry about where her legs were and what they were doing.

What he explained to us was that the real risk was that if her legs were in the stirrups and she moved the wrong way, she could break a hip very easily. So there we were, I was on one side, Jennifer was on the other side and we held her legs back as far as we could without hurting her. Out came the first baby, fairly easily; she just slipped right out.

Mind you, by this point I had thrown my video camera on the couch. The doctor turned to Jennifer and I and asked, "Who's going to cut the cord?" We had no idea we were going to be this involved. It was wonderful. Jennifer didn't say anything, so I volunteered. I cut the cord of our baby girl, Katherine. They whisked her away to the little incubator, cleaned her up.

Then the doctor told Brittany to relax. She needed to give it a little bit of time before the second baby could come. As the second baby was crowning, the doctor had to tell Brittany not to push because there was a risk that she could tear herself and there was no point in doing that. She had to relax and let the baby naturally slide out on his own, and he did. By this point, we knew that someone was going to cut his cord, and I wasn't going to get to cut both of them, so Jennifer cut Christopher's cord. I grabbed the camera and took a picture of that, which was a wonderful moment.

They cleaned him up and both were admitted to the NICU, which is special care for infants that are born early. Our children were born seven weeks early so they were quite premature; however, they were, as we call it, the biggest babies on the block. Katherine weighed 6lbs. 2oz. at birth and Christopher weighed 5lbs. 9oz. Most preemies weigh less than four pounds and often two to three pounds, depending on how early they are, especially twins.

We felt very blessed to have such big babies. That can give you a false sense of security; however, because although they were big and looked very healthy, their internal organs were still immature, so they spent 19 days in the NICU.

Post-Birth

Brittany was discharged the very next day, after having the babies. The same week she was discharged, we got a call from her while we were at the NICU visiting our children. She said she was in great pain. Brittany's sister had taken her children to their grandparents' house so Brittany was at the house by herself. She called and said she had to go to the emergency room because the pain was just so great.

We were conflicted because we were saying, "We're here with our babies." I didn't want to go. I wanted her to call someone else or a cab or have her drive herself. I felt that our relationship was pretty well over at this point. But we certainly felt a sense of obligation and duty to continue to be there for her because we knew she didn't have anybody else at that moment.

I went and Jennifer stayed at the hospital with the babies. I picked her up and took her to the OBGYN. We weren't sure what was going on, so he prescribed some medication for her and a urology appointment for a week later, which was the earliest we could get.

Brittany and I left the hospital, and went to pick up Jennifer. Part of our documentary was being shot at the hospital, which is why we were at the hospital and why Jennifer had to stay, because the film crew and producers were there.

When I arrived, everything wasn't finished yet, so we asked Brittany to wait in the private waiting room while we finished up. While she was out there, she got sick and vomited and just wasn't feeling good at all. Finally, we had to wrap it up.

Rush-Hour in Atlanta

We were in rush hour traffic. We'd only gone two exits, and it took us 30 minutes. Brittany was still in extreme pain. I decided to turn back around and get her back to the emergency room, because there was no way she was going home. I knew what it meant if I didn't take her back. It meant that at 3:00 o'clock in the morning, I'd be getting up and taking her to the emergency room anyway, so I wanted to do it now.

Not only did she need it, but also, I was thinking about us. We took her back. She was admitted and actually had more gallstones to pass. We stayed with her at the hospital. This was a week after the babies were born. Our babies were in the hospital, so we were up at the hospital with her.

She spoke with her mother and she shared with us that her mother had told her to stop relying on the parents and encouraged her to move back to the city where she was from. That was the first indication that our relationship may be changing, from one of dependence to one of, let's regain our own identities and independence again. That was difficult, as well.

The House and Brittany

Both she and we had intended to continue renting the house that we had purchased. It was completely paid for on our end, so we didn't have any hard costs, but Jennifer and I had made the decision that Jennifer would be a stay at home mother and would stop working and that meant part of our income was now gone.

While we thought we were going to be able to afford that situation, I'm an independent business owner. After the babies were born in March of 2010, I experienced a slump in my business, which could have probably been predicted because I was spending all of my time at the hospital with the babies. If you're not in your business running it, it does not run.

So for the very first time, my motherly instincts of do or die kicked in. I thought, "We're going to lose everything financially. We've spent everything we've got; we created this family, and now I'm feeling a crunch, and we're going to lose everything that we've got." It was a very difficult decision and discussion to have with our surrogate, who we knew was depending on us, to say we have to sell the home you live in. We needed her to move out.

A Fork in the Road

When we had that discussion, we had intended to do it in person but it wasn't working out for whatever reason. I had to email her, which may be the most common form of communication today but was not the best form of communication to deal with sensitive issues.

We received an email back. I felt very fortunate that she felt comfortable enough to share her opinions and feelings with us. She said, in so many words, that she felt abandoned. She said, "I don't have a home or job; I have two children and I don't know what to do or where to go."

We found ourselves at a fork in the road. Should we take care of our own family or take care of someone else's family, a woman who had done so much for us? What we had done was to support her emotionally as much as we possibly could through the transition. We certainly weren't able to change our mind and say, "Oh, I didn't know you would feel that way. Why don't you stay?" This would have meant risking our financial future, to include the house Brittany lived in.

Keeping in Touch

We continued to support Brittany emotionally. She did move back to her hometown. She did get work to support herself and her children and things have gone back to, basically, the way they were before we met and had children. We do stay in touch. We continue to send pictures and she sends updates on what's going on in her life. So, now, we have another person in our life that is very important to us but there is a sense of saying goodbye and carrying on a relationship in a different way.

In Closing
• • • • • • • • • •

"Children are the world's most valuable resource and its best hope for the future."

—*John Fitzgerald Kennedy*

But, the most important people of all in this story are Katherine and Christopher, our two beautiful babies. All the time, energy, and money we expended during the almost five years we spent getting to baby seem so worth it now. However, our goal is to help others reduce the amount of time, energy, and money they spend before getting to baby. Because it can be done. Being parents is the most rewarding "job" we've ever had—watching them grow and change and learn new things every day. The first time they roll over, sit up, crawl, laugh, give you a big wet open mouthed kiss. We are about to celebrate their first birthday and the last year has been more fun than we could have ever imagined.

YOU can do it too—faster, easier, and less expensive. We have witnessed other couples create their families in 12 months or less using artificial insemination, IVF, adoption, and surrogacy. Follow the guidance in Getting to Baby, and you WILL create your family. For more information, updated regularly, go to our website, www.GettingtoBaby.com.

Our experience using a surrogate was rewarding on many levels. Regardless of the path you choose, we wish you all the best and will be with you in our thoughts and prayers.

About the Authors

Victoria Collier lives in Georgia where she has her own law practice helping the elderly. She is a published author, national speaker, and veteran of the United States Air Force. Victoria has a most loving dog, Joey, who is smitten with the children.

Jennifer Collier is a twin herself. She was a prosecutor for 15 years prior to becoming a mother. Jennifer now stays home with the children; her most challenging and rewarding job to date.

Victoria and Jennifer met in South Georgia in 1997. They knew from the beginning they wanted to have children together. Embarking on this journey has been one to both challenge and strengthen their relationship.

Jennifer and Christopher (left), Victoria and Katherine (right) outside our home in a suburb of Atlanta, Georgia.

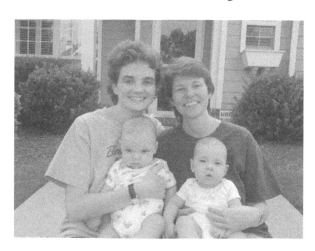

BONUS OFFER

Thank you for reading Getting to Baby.

It is our mission to help as many couples as possible achieve their dreams of having children. For more helpful information, go to our website, www.GettingtoBaby.com.

Your FREE Bonus Offer—*Creating a Family in the 21st Century Documovie*—is accessible on our website, www.GettingtoBaby.com by entering PROMO Code: JTCK.

We encourage you to send us your story and join us on the community forum at www.GettingtoBaby.com, where others are sharing their experiences.

BUY A SHARE OF THE FUTURE IN YOUR COMMUNITY

These certificates make great holiday, graduation and birthday gifts that can be personalized with the recipient's name. The cost of one S.H.A.R.E. or one square foot is $54.17. The personalized certificate is suitable for framing and will state the number of shares purchased and the amount of each share, as well as the recipient's name. The home that you participate in "building" will last for many years and will continue to grow in value.

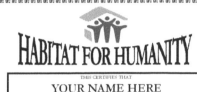

THIS CERTIFIES THAT

YOUR NAME HERE

HAS INVESTED IN A HOME FOR A DESERVING FAMILY

1985-2010

TWENTY-FIVE YEARS OF BUILDING FUTURES
IN OUR COMMUNITY ONE HOME AT A TIME

1200 SQUARE FOOT HOUSE @ $65,900 = $54.17 PER SQUARE FOOT
This certificate represents a tax deductible donation. It has no cash value.

Here is a sample SHARE certificate:

YES, I WOULD LIKE TO HELP!

I support the work that Habitat for Humanity does and I want to be part of the excitement! As a donor, I will receive periodic updates on your construction activities but, more importantly, I know my gift will help a family in our community realize the dream of homeownership. **I would like to SHARE in your efforts against substandard housing in my community!** *(Please print below)*

PLEASE SEND ME _____ SHARES at $54.17 EACH = $ $_____

In Honor Of: _____

Occasion: (Circle One)   HOLIDAY   BIRTHDAY   ANNIVERSARY

        OTHER: _____

Address of Recipient: _____

Gift From: _____   *Donor Address:* _____

Donor Email: _____

I AM ENCLOSING A CHECK FOR $ $_____ PAYABLE TO HABITAT FOR HUMANITY OR PLEASE CHARGE MY VISA OR MASTERCARD *(CIRCLE ONE)*

Card Number _____   Expiration Date: _____

Name as it appears on Credit Card _____   Charge Amount $ _____

Signature _____

Billing Address _____

Telephone # Day _____   Eve _____

PLEASE NOTE: Your contribution is tax-deductible to the fullest extent allowed by law.
Habitat for Humanity • P.O. Box 1443 • Newport News, VA 23601 • 757-596-5553
www.HelpHabitatforHumanity.org

Printed in the USA
CPSIA information can be obtained
at www.ICGtesting.com
JSHW022335140824
68134JS00019B/1505

9 780982 859094